MANUAL OF ANAESTHESIA FOR SMALL ANIMAL PRACTICE

(Third Revised Edition)

Edited by

A. D. R. Hilbery
B.Vet.Med., M.R.C.V.S.

assisted by

A. E. Waterman
B.V.Sc., Ph.D., D.V.A., M.R.C.V.S.

G. J. Brouwer
B. Vet. Med., B.Sc., D.V.A., M.R.C.V.S.

Published by the
British Small Animal
Veterinary Association
Kingsley House, Church Lane,
Shurdington, Cheltenham,
Gloucestershire GL51 5TQ

Printed by KCO, Worthing
West Sussex.

Copyright BSAVA 1989. All rights reserved.
No part of this publication may be
reproduced, stored in a retrieval
system or transmitted in any form
or by any means electronic, mechanical,
photocopying, recording or otherwise
without prior permission of the
copyright owner.

The publisher cannot take any responsibility
for information provided on dosages and methods
of application of drugs mentioned in this publication.
Details of this kind must be verified by individual users
in the appropriate literature.

First Published 1989
Third Revised Edition 1992

ISBN 0 905214 09 9

CONTENTS

Contents .... 2 & 3
Acknowledgements 5
Foreword 7

Chapter One
    General Principles of Anaesthesia 9
      L. W. Hall

Chapter Two
    **Pre-operative Assessment,
    Monitoring and Post-operative Care** 17
      P. M. Taylor

Chapter Three
    Anaesthetic Equipment and Safety 25
      R. S. Jones

Chapter Four
    Analgesia 33
      A. M. Nolan

Chapter Five
    Premedication and Sedation 39
      K. W. Clarke

Chapter Six
    Intravenous Anaesthesia 51
      A. E. Waterman, J. N. Lucke

Chapter Seven
    Inhalation Anaesthesia 65
      R. S. Jones

Chapter Eight
    Local Anaesthesia 75
      K. W. Clarke

CONTENTS

Chapter Nine
Use of Muscle Relaxants 83
G. J. Brouwer

Chapter Ten
Anaesthesia for Caesarian Section 87
B. M. Q. Weaver

Chapter Eleven
Anaesthesia for Thoracic Surgery 95
G. J. Brouwer

Chapter Twelve
Anaesthesia for Ophthalmic Surgery 101
B. M. Q. Weaver

Chapter Thirteen
Anaesthesia of Geriatrics and Neonates 107
A. E. Waterman

Chapter Fourteen
Anaesthesia in High Risk Cases 113
A. E. Waterman

Chapter Fifteen
Fluid Therapy 119
J. C. Brearley

Chapter Sixteen
Anaesthetic Accidents and Emergencies 129
D. L. S. Richards

Chapter Seventeen
Anaesthesia of Exotic Species 139
J. E. Cooper

Appendix 152
Index 154
B.S.A.V.A. Publications 156

ACKNOWLEDGEMENTS

I would like to express my thanks to The Association of Veterinary Anaesthetists of Great Britain, of which all the authors are members and especially to Avril Waterman and Gerard Brouwer, the editorial board, for their help, advice and support.

As always, Michael Gorton Design, our trusted typesetters have been indefatigable. Without their guidance deadlines would have certainly been missed and the Manual would not have had its attractive layout. Millie Gorton has been a tower of strength and has always produced chapters and returned proofs even more quickly than asked.

The addition of an index will, I think, make the book easier to use and thanks are due to B. V. Martin Associates for carrying out the indexing, a task from which I shrank.

Finally, I would like to thank my wife, Jane and my children for their forbearance on all those evenings when I was poring over 'The Book' and wasn't able to help with homework or even be sociable.

A. D. R. Hilbery,
Hawthorn Hill Cottage,
February 1989

FOREWORD

The concept of the BSAVA Manual is now well established. It fills a specific need in practice for a succinct text, logically laid out enabling rapid reference and immediate understanding. The world of veterinary science moves ahead at a rapid pace and at its forefront is anaesthesiology.

This is the third edition of this Manual in ten years, which reflects both the need to include 'state-of-the-art' information and how appropriate this format is in permitting such frequent text adjustment, addition or complete rewriting. I welcome this forthright approach as a general practitioner. Additionally, as President, I am gratified by the enthusiasm of the eleven authors to this text and I am grateful for Publications Committee work in putting it together.

'For a ha'peth of tar the ship was lost' can be annotated to the techniques to produce balanced and safe anaethesia. Surgery without good anaesthesia is nothing. The glamour of the former is ephemeral without a static and malleable surgical field.

Anaesthesiology itself has had its static times. There have been occasions of startling advance and innovation and then, cyclically, moments of quiescence almost retrenchment. This is one such time of advance. New equipment and improved techniques abound. The safety considerations for patient and operator are an immediate consideration. The arrival of new compounds provides the anaesthetist, as never before, with a multiplicity of choice; such that simple procedures requiring restraint need carry only the smallest risk factor. All of these points are addressed in this new manual.

The veterinary surgeon must be academically malleable. Unlike most sister professions, the demands placed on us vary according to an economic turn or a human fancy. Witness the ever increasing interest in exotic species, pedigree animals, and the improved expectation from owners. All demand a quick-footedness in knowledge and expertise. Consistent results are looked for in the anaesthesia of neonates and geriatric animals, for caesarians and in complicated procedures such as thoracic and cardiovascular surgery and in shock states.

This book does not set out to be a comprehensive dissertation on small animal anaesthesia but rather, as Tony Hilbery said in his preface to the second edition in 1984: "it was envisaged as a daily guide for use in general practice, a book that will be ready to hand and easy to refer to". The authors, members of the Association of Veterinary Anaesthetists are to be commended for achieving just that. As a mark of our appreciation, the BSAVA is delighted to have made a contribution to the AVA Educational Trust.

John Foster, BVSc., Cert.V.Ophthal., MRCVS.,
President, BSAVA

FOREWORD TO THIRD (Revised) EDITION

Such has been the success of this Manual that it has sold out well before the end of its useful life. We would normally expect to produce a new edition about every four to five years, and that time has not come yet. However, there have been some significant advances and changes since 1989, mainly in the fields of Alpha 2 Adrenoceptor Agonists and of safety; especially in the light of the COSHH regulations.

This revised edition, therefore, mostly corrects previous errors and makes minor revisions, with two very important exceptions. In her chapter on Premedication and Sedation, Dr. K. W. Clarke has given an update of current knowledge and applications of the α 2 Adrenoceptor Agonists and Antagonists, with special reference to Medetomidine and Atipamezole. Secondly, M. H. Clark has written an appendix on safety, scavenging and COSHH regulations.

These two additions alone make the manual more appropriate for the present. The potent actions of Medetomidine and its antagonist Atipamezole are powerful weapons in the armamentarium of veterinary anaesthetists, but it behoves us to use them with caution. Dr. Clarke sets all this out very clearly in her chapter.

The appendix on safety is timely indeed and will, I think, make startling reading. I know that it has made me think seriously about the precautions that we should be taking for the protection of ourselves and our staff.

I would like to thank the Authors for their rapid response to my request for revisions and corrections and also Brian Hamblett of Michael Gorton Design for his help and patience when asked at very short notice to insert a completely new section.

A.D.R.H.
February 1992

CHAPTER 1

GENERAL PRINCIPLES OF ANAESTHESIA

L. W. Hall M.A., B.Sc., Ph.D., D.V.A., M.R.C.V.S.

THE NEED FOR ANAESTHESIA

HUMANITARIAN

Animals' perception of pain must be inferred but so must the mental states of our fellow human beings; there is no anatomical, philosophical or psysiological reason for denying that man and animals perceive pain in much the same way. Humane considerations must always be uppermost in the veterinarian's approach to animals and every effort should be made to prevent what would, in man, constitute suffering.

TECHNICAL EFFICIENCY

In small animal practice, anaesthesia can be so safe that it may be employed simply as a means of restraint, even when no pain is involved (e.g. to produce immobility for radiography). Many procedures are greatly facilitated by relaxation of skeletal muscles, whilst others can only be performed when the lungs of the anaesthetised animal are being artificially ventilated.

LEGAL OBLIGATION

In many countries, including the U.K., there is a legal obligation imposed on veterinarians to adopt effective measures for the prevention of suffering during the performance of pain-provoking procedures. All veterinarians must be familiar with the relevant legislation of the country in which they work.

The guidelines for veterinarians in the U.K. provided by the Registrar of the Royal College of Veterinary Surgeons, emphasise:-

Duty of Care.

The veterinarian has a duty of care towards the client in deciding whether anaesthesia can safely be undertaken; a duty of care in deciding upon the appropriate form of anaesthesia; a duty of care in the administration of the anaesthetic and a duty of care in consultation with any other veterinarians involved in the case of ensuring that the client is properly advised regarding the course to be followed and any special notes involved. As always, the veterinarian must also 'bring to his task a reasonable degree of skill and knowledge and must exercise a reasonable degree of care'. Failure to do so, which results in the death or injury of an animal, gives the owner the right to bring legal action for recovery of damages.

Negligence.

An error of judgement does not **necessarily** amount to negligence. Whether or not the requisite degree of competence, skill and knowledge has been exercised in any particular case is normally tested against what is seen to be normal, currently accepted practice.

It is the duty of the veterinary anaesthetist to be sure that anyone asked to assist with anaesthesia of an animal is competent to perform the tasks assigned to them. Failure to do so may constitute negligence.

AIMS OF ANAESTHESIA

1. To prevent awareness of pain.
2. To provide immobility of the patient and when required relaxation of the skeletal muscles.
3. To achieve the above without jeopardising the safety of the animal during the operation or the pre- and post-operative periods.

All these aims can sometimes be achieved by the administration of a single agent. More commonly, drugs having a nearly single, specific action in the body are combined to ensure safe and pleasant anaesthesia. Very occasionally, the safety of the animal cannot be safeguarded while the other aims are achieved, without the surgeon accepting some degree of inconvenience.

METHODS OF ANAESTHESIA

GENERAL ANAESTHESIA

Any method of preventing awareness of pain which involves loss of consciousness and inability to recall events associated with a procedure, constitutes 'general anaesthesia'. It normally involves a process of controlled, reversible intoxication of the central nervous system.

General anaesthesia is usually produced by the administration of 'narcotic drugs' which produce unconsciousness and an absence of motor response to noxious stimuli; all anaesthetics are narcotics but not all narcotics are anaesthetics. (Note that: 'narcotic' in statutory legislation usually means a drug of human addiction.) Acupuncture is not generally regarded as acceptable for routine use and attempts to anaesthetise animals by passing controlled electric currents through the skull or vertebral column have met with little success.

General anaesthesia may be:-

Inhalational.

Where the agents are administered in the respired gases. Although some metabolism may occur, these agents are mainly excreted unchanged through the lungs. Elimination from the inspired gases, coupled with artificial ventilation, usually removes them from the body quickly so that resuscitation following inadvertent overdose is simple; inhalation anaesthesia is, therefore, generally regarded as very safe.

The alveolar concentration of the agent which abolishes movement in response to a painful stimulus in 50% of animals (minimal alveolar concentration, MAC), has been determined for all the commonly used anaesthetics. Knowledge of this value allows very safe use of volatile anaesthetic agents when non-rebreathing systems are used in conjunction with accurately calibrated vaporisers.

Intravenous.

Where the agent is injected directly into the bloodstream either as a bolus or by slow infusion. Once administered, the agent cannot be recovered from the body and elimination depends on detoxification and/or excretion (mainly in the bile or urine). Safety depends on strict control of the dose administered and what might constitute a safe dose for a normal, young, healthy animal, may be a gross overdose for an elderly or ill animal. Overdose can be fatal in the absence of apparatus for respiratory resuscitation and the administration of oxygen. Recovery is primarily determined by the kinetic profiles of the drugs used and, if they are rapidly cleared from the body, can sometimes be faster than after inhalation anaesthesia.

At any time during the procedure, the amount of anaesthetic actually given to the patient can be known with certainty. Experience of how similar cases have behaved with similar doses, enables fairly accurate forecasting of the outcome to be made.

The use of intravenous agents eliminates the possible hazards of exposure of personnel to trace concentrations of volatile and gaseous anaesthetic agents.

LOCAL ANALGESIA

Local analgesia follows from temporary, peripheral blockade of sensory nerves. Local analgesic drugs may have undesirable or even dangerous effects after absorption from their site of application.

Topical application.
Has limited use, being confined to the conjunctiva and the mucous membranes of the nose, pharynx, tracheobronchial tree, penis, vagina, rectum and urethra; the drugs are applied as drops of solution, a spray, or in a carboxymethylcellulose gel.

Infiltration and regional block analgesia.
Produced by injection. Infiltration analgesia is produced by injection into the operation site; regional blocks are accomplished by injection around nerve trunks supplying sensation to the region.

Epidural analgesia.
Produced in dogs and cats by the injection of drugs usually at the lumbo-sacral space. Its usefulness is limited by the complications arising from a temporarily paraplegic animal.

Intravenous regional analgesia.
May be produced by the intravenous injection of drugs distal to the site of an arterial tourniquet. Analgesia develops quickly and lasts as long as the tourniquet produces ischaemia.

CHOICE OF ANAESTHETIC METHOD

This is influenced by:-

The facilities available.
Intravenous barbiturates given with care may be safer than a poorly administered inhalation anaesthetic given with inappropriate apparatus.

The skill and experience of the anaesthetist and surgeon.
And whether the anaesthetic is to be administered by a surgeon/anaesthetist with intra-operative supervision from a nurse.

The facilities for post-operative care.
The need to return an animal to its owner for post-operative nursing may mean that local analgesia or a general anaesthetic with a short recovery period should be used. Careful thought must always be given to the provision of post-operative pain relief in these cases.

The temperament of the patient.
In good natured dogs and cats sedative premedication may be unnecessary before the induction of anaesthesia with an intravenous agent. Some cats may be so unmanageable that anaesthesia has to be induced by confining them in a small box and introducing an inhalation agent into the box. Vigorous or vicious dogs may require strong restraint for the administration of heavy sedative premedication before anaesthesia.

The species and breed of the animal.
Dogs should not be given anaesthetic agents containing the solubiliser 'Cremophor EL'. Some breeds respond badly to drugs which may be used freely in other breeds.

The age and health of the animal.
Old age and ill health usually call for reduction of the doses of anaesthetic drugs rather than drastic alteration of technique. Suckling puppies and kittens should not be given parenteral agents and the provision of warmth to maintain body temperature is essential for all elderly and young animals.

The vast majority of animals suffering from disease can be safely anaesthetised after proper pre-anaesthetic preparation. Infections should be treated with antimicrobials, diabetes mellitis should be controlled and fluid balance disturbances should be corrected. Every effort must be made to see that the animal is as fit as practicable before it is anaesthetised.

The site of operation.

Operations on the head or neck, oral and dental surgery are indications for endotracheal intubation. Oral or dental surgery necessitates packing of the pharynx to prevent accumulation of blood and debris that may be inhaled after extubation at the end of the procedure. Bronchoscopy presents problems because the bronchoscopist works in the airway and different anaesthetic techniques may be needed for fibre-optic compared with rigid bronchoscope instrumentation. Intrathoracic surgery compels the use of endotracheal intubation and intermittent positive pressure ventilation of the lungs. In dogs, intra-abdominal surgery is greatly facilitated by the muscle relaxation produced by epidural block or relaxant drugs.

The nature of the operation.

Caesarian section requires the administration of minimal quantities of premedicant and general anaesthetic drugs or the use of some form of local analgesia. Vaginal delivery may be possible with no more than mild sedation. Oral surgery, dental surgery and operations about the airway, demand a rapid return of protective reflexes post-operatively. Examinations under anaesthesia (e.g. radiography) often need little more than a short period of immobility followed by a rapid return of consciousness. Anaesthesia for these examinations are often major undertakings; there may be 'minor' procedures but never 'minor' anaesthetics.

The duration of the operation.

Minor, short procedures such as removal of grass awns from the aural canal, may be performed after the intravenous injection of thiopentone, methohexitone or propofol.

When periods of anaesthesia greater than three to four minutes are needed for minor procedures, unpremedicated cats and dogs may be anaesthetised with propofol and further doses of this agent given as required. Cats and some smaller pets, may be anaesthetised with 'Saffan' in a similar manner. For most major surgery and for prolonged procedures, anaesthesia may be induced with an intravenous agent and maintained with an inhalation anaesthetic or an infusion of the intravenous agent used for induction.

ANAESTHETIC/PREPARATION/RECOVERY ROOMS

As far as possible animals should be prepared for operation (clipped, shaved, washed, given enemata, etc.) before anaesthesia is induced. Preparation after induction greatly increases the duration of anaesthesia and the risk of complications, especially in animals suffering from cardiovascular or respiratory disease. Most animals can be prepared after premedication has taken effect and because preparation is a non-sterile procedure, it is best carried out in the kennel area, away from surgical facilities. Excessive wetting of the animal must be avoided since it may give rise to hypothermia.

An anaesthetic/recovery area adjacent to the operating theatre is highly desirable. All anaesthetic equipment can be kept there, ready to hand. After anaesthesia, animals can be kept in the recovery area under close observation, until judged fit to return to the kennel accommodation. Crises in the immediate post-operative period can be detected and dealt with promptly since the necessary equipment is ready at hand.

The dimensions of the anaesthetic room/recovery area should be decided in the light of the anaesthetic and surgical work loads. The design and layout may be dictated by existing structures but thought should be given to aspects of traffic flow for patients, trolleys and staff. A small basin for a detergent/disinfectant solution in which endotracheal tubes, face masks, etc., may be soaked after use prior to cleaning, is most desirable. Hand-washing facilities must be provided and the lighting of the area requires attention. If fluorescent lights are fitted, care should be taken to install correct tube types so that colour distortion, which causes difficulty in assessing the colour of mucous membranes, does not occur.

Good storage space for syringes, endotracheal tubes, breathing circuits and drugs, must be provided and an adequate work surface is essential. Modern kitchen furniture is admirably suited for these purposes. Room ventilation must be carefully considered and proper arrangements made for ducting waste anaesthetic gases and vapours out of the anaesthetic area.

In the recovery areas, animals are best nursed on trolleys with low, open mesh sides to give maximum accessibility for essential nursing care. Oxygen tents and cages may limit access to the patient; when necessary, oxygen can be administered by face-mask or naso-pharyngeal catheter.

PERSONNEL

Well trained nursing staff can do much to relieve the veterinarian from some of the routine aspects of anaesthesia. Washing, cleaning and sterilisation of equipment and its preparation for use should be all the responsibility of the nursing staff.

Induction of anaesthesia and its termination should always be carried out by, or under the direct supervision of, a veterinarian, but a suitably trained nurse may administer premedication and monitor the patient's condition during an operation, administering drugs or adjusting a vaporiser control on the direct instruction of the veterinarian in charge.

A well trained nurse should be able to perform endotracheal intubation in unconscious or anaesthetised animals, carry out intermittent positive pressure ventilation (I.P.P.V.), set up intravenous infusions, give subcutaneous, intramuscular and intravenous injections and pass uninary catheters. The nurse should also be taught to recognise the signs of respiratory depression, respiratory obstruction and haemorrhage, which are most likely to occur in the immediate post-anaesthetic period.

EQUIPMENT

Continuous flow anaesthetic machine with gas supply (see Chapter 3).

Cylinder keys.

Anaesthetic breathing circuits.

> **Essential:** T-piece system and Magill (Mapleson A System) or Bain Circuit (Penlon Ltd., Abingdon OX14 3PH) or Lack circuit (MIE Ltd. Falcon Road, Sowton Industrial Estate, Exeter, Devon).
>
> **Optional:** Non-rebreathing valves (e.g. Ambu, Ruben's), carbon dioxide absorber circuits (To-and-fro Waters' system or circle system).

Face Masks.
Sizes: large (dog), medium (dog) and small (cat).

Endotracheal tubes.
Red rubber or plastic.
Suggested sizes: up to 5mm internal diameter plain, from 5.5mm to 16mm internal diameter, cuffed.

Endotracheal tube connectors.
To fit directly to breathing circuit (Portex Plastics or Bowring Engineering, 31 Quarry Road, Witney, Oxford).

Laryngoscope.
With adult and infant size Soper blades (Penlon Ltd., Abindon OX14 3PH).

Suction apparatus.
With metal and plastic suction catheters.

Stethoscope.
Chestpiece and oesophageal.

Syringes.
2ml, 5ml, 10ml and 20ml (5ml, 10ml and 20ml should have side nozzles).

Needles.

1.2 x 40mm (18 swg x 1½")   0.8 x 25mm (21 swg x 1")
0.6 x 25mm (23 swg x 1")   0.5 x 16mm (25 swg x 5/8")

Miscellaneous Equipment

Scissors (curved on flat)

Galley pots and receivers (preferably aluminium foil or paper mache and disposable)

Electric hair clippers.

Vacuum cleaner.

Waste bin with lid.

Small sand bags, bean bags sealed in plastic envelopes or radiolucent plastic body supports.

Tape muzzles and restraining tapes.

Gauze swabs.

Adhesive plaster.

KY Jelly and lignocaine ointment or urethral gel.

Ancillary Equipment

Doppler-shift flow detector with sphygmomanometer.

Esmarch's bandages and rubber tubing tourniquets.

Electrical thermometer with a large dial together with rectal and nasopharyngeal probes.

Fluid administration sets, plastic, disposable, with and without filters.

Drip extension tubes or manometer lines (disposable).

Disposable 3-way stopcocks.

Intravenous cannulae and catheters, disposable, cannula — or catheter-over-needle types.

Electrolyte and other intravenous infusions. Minimum:-
    Dextrose saline solution.
    Hartmann's solution (Comp. Sod. Lact. Inj. BP) and a plasma volume expander such as 'Haemaccel' or 'Gelofusin'.

Urethral catheters, male catheters and Foley catheters with introducers.

Anaesthetic record charts.

Maintenance Equipment

Screwdrivers, including Phillips screwdriver.

Set of spanners up to ½" Whitworth.

Set of hexagonal wrenches (Allen keys) British and metric sizes.

Wooden mallet.

Spare cylinder washers.

Spare laryngoscope bulbs.

DRUGS

The choice of drugs is largely governed by personal preference of the anaesthetist but most needs should be met by:-

    Atropine (1ml ampoules containing 0.6mg atropine).

    Glycopyrrolate ('Robinul Injectable', A. H. Robins, 20ml multidose bottle 0.2 mg/ml).

    Acepromazine (multidose bottle, 2 mg/ml).

    Ketamine hydrochloride ('Vetalar', Parke-Davis).

    Morphine (ampoules of 10 mg).

    Pethidine Hydrochloride (ampoules of 100 mg).

    Buprenorphine
        ('Temgesic', Reckitt & Coleman, 1 ml ampoules containing 0.3 mg buprenorphine).

    Diazepam ('Diazemuls', 10 mg ampoules).

    Thiopentone sodium (2.5 gramme containers with 100 ml of water to prepare a 2.5% solution).

    Methohexitone sodium (usually used as a 1% or 2% solution).

    Propofol ('Rapinovet', Cooper's Animal Health).

    Alphaxalone with alphadolone ('Saffan', Pitman Moore).

    Halothane.

    Methoxyflurane.

    Enflurane.

    Isoflurane.

    Suxamethonium. ('Brevidil', R.M.B., 'Scoline', Duncan, Flockhart, 'Anectine' Calmic).

    Pancuronium bromide 'Pavulon', Organon-Teknika).

    Vecuronium bromide ('Norcuron', Organon-Teknika).

    Atracurium besylate ('Tracrium' Burroughs Wellcome).

    Neostigmine hydrobromide ('Prostigmine', Roche).

    Lignocaine hydrochloride (1% solution without vasoconstrictor).

    Adrenaline hydrochloride (1 ml ampoules of 1:1000).

    Isoprenaline.

    Naloxone ('Narcan', 0.4 mg/ml, Winthrop Laboratories).

    Sodium bicarbonate (ampoules 2.5%).

    Ergometrine tartrate (ampoules of 0.125 and 0.5 mg/ml).

Other Drugs

    Alfentanil (Janssen Pharmaceutica).

    Fentanyl ('Sublimaze', Janssen Pharmaceutica).

    Fluanisone-fentanyl ('Hypnorm' Janssen Pharmaceutica).

    Xylazine ('Rompun', Bayer).

    Heparin (to make up heparinized saline solution).

    Medetomidine (SmithKline Beecham).

    Atipamezole (SmithKline Beecham).

CHAPTER 2   # PRE-OPERATIVE ASSESSMENT, MONITORING AND POST-OPERATIVE CARE

P. M. Taylor M.A., Vet.M.B., Ph.D., D.V.A., M.R.C.V.S.

PREOPERATIVE ASSESSMENT

Many veterinary operations are carried out on normal healthy patients and death under anaesthesia can usually be attributed to human error. It is essential that every animal is examined before sedation or anaesthesia in order to ensure that they are normal or to detect abnormalities which will necessitate special treatment before or during anaesthesia.

The anaesthetic risk is dependent upon both the condition of the patient and the facilities and expertise available. Some classification of the patient's condition is a helpful aid to assessment of anaesthetic risk and the American Society of Anesthesiologists' system provides a useful guide:

Class 1. A normal healthy patient.
Class 2. A patient with mild systemic disease.
Class 3. A patient with severe systemic disease that is not incapacitating.
Class 4. A patient with severe systemic disease that is a constant threat to life.
Class 5. A moribund patient not expected to survive for 24 hours with or without operation.

Emergency cases are classified by the addition of 'E' to the number. An emergency case carries greater risk both as a result of the presenting condition and because preoperative tests and preparation are curtailed.

The patient's preoperative condition is assessed from the history and a clinical examination.

HISTORY

concurrent drug therapy: eg corticosteroids, NSAIDs, antibiotics, cardiac glycosides and beta blockers may interact with anaesthetic drugs.

poor exercise tolerance and breathlessness: may indicate cardiac or respiratory disease.

cough: moist cough indicates presence of airway secretions, harsh cough may indicate chronic airway disease.

polydipsia and polyuria: may indicate renal disease.

vomiting and diarrhoea: may be gastro intestinal or other systemic disease, likely to have fluid and electrolyte deficits.

inappetance: common with infectious disease and painful conditions.

time of last meal: to assess risk of vomiting. Elective surgery should not be performed on animals which have been fed within the last six hours.

history of any previous anaesthetics or sedations: an untoward reaction may indicate that a different technique should be used on this occasion.

history of any abnormal behaviour (eg convulsions): drugs which reduce the convulsive threshold (such as phenothiazines) should be avoided.

breed: some breeds have a reputation for adverse or exaggerated responses to anaesthesia. Boxers and the very large breeds are profoundly affected by relatively small doses of the phenothiazines.

CLINICAL EXAMINATION

Inspection

deformities especially of head and neck, condition of teeth and mouth and ease of opening mouth: all may affect intubation and maintenance of airway.

colour of mucous membranes: pale, suggests hypovolaemia or anaemia. Cyanotic, indicates sluggish circulation or poor oxygenation of arterial blood.

brightness of eyes and coat, degree of mental alertness: indication of general health.

respiratory pattern: tachypnoea, may indicate respiratory or cardiac disease or excitement and fear. Dyspnoea indicates respiratory disease.

obesity: puts cardiovascular system under greater stress.

jugular venous filling: increased right atrial or ventricular pressure, may indicate chronic lung disease.

Palpation

pulse: increased rate or weak and thready quality may indicate excitement and fear, hypovolaemia or myocardial insufficiency.

dryness of mouth and skin turgor: dry mouth and poor skin turgor indicates hypovolaemia, water and electrolyte deficit. Oedema suggests hypoproteinaemia or cardiac insufficiency.

lymph nodes: increased size suggests infection or neoplasia.

chest movement: inequality of the two sides suggests pulmonary or pleural disease.

cardiac apex beat: abnormal position suggests space occupying lesion in thorax.

vascular thrills: suggest cardiovascular abnormality.

palpate for evidence of pain.

Percussion

comparison of resonance over chest walls: areas of low resonance suggest consolidated lung, fluid or space occupying lesion. High resonance is found with pneumothorax.

Auscultation

respiratory system: adventitious sounds indicate airway secretion or respiratory disease. Reduced or absent sounds indicate consolidation or a space occupying lesion.

heart: a systolic murmur may or may not be significant. A diastolic murmur always indicates heart disease. Dysrhythmias (other than sinus arhythmia with respiration) indicate heart disease.

Special tests

haematology: for haemoglobin and leucocyte picture.

biochemistry: urea and creatinine for kidney function, liver function tests and enzymes for liver function, urinalysis for kidney function (ability to concentrate).

radiography: for investigation of respiratory and cardiac disease.

ECG: for investigation of dysrhythmias.

SIGNIFICANCE OF FINDINGS

Respiratory disease

Restricted airway (eg nasal discharge, bulldog anatomy): requires particular attention to maintenance of the airway during anaesthesia and in the recovery period. Pulmonary disease should be further investigated with radiography before anaesthesia. Pleural effusion should be drained before anaesthesia.

Cardiac disease

The heart's ability to pump effectively is more important than the nature of the heart disease. Fitness for anaesthesia is largely related to exercise tolerance. Any condition which limits the heart's ability to increase output under stress is life threatening.

Renal disease

Renal failure increases the risk of anaesthesia as uraemia markedly increases sensitivity to anaesthetic drugs and any renal drug excretion is reduced. Uraemia should be corrected by fluid infusion before anaesthesia. Development of uraemia may be prevented in animals with chronic renal failure by fluid infusion during anaesthesia.

Hypovolaemia and anaemia

Fluid deficits, whatever their cause, should be corrected as far as possible before anaesthesia (see chapter 15). Anaemia, unless very severe (haemoglobin below 5 gm/dL or haematocrit below 0.2 L/L) is not a serious hazard as long as high inspired oxygen tensions are provided to ensure the blood carries as much oxygen as possible. An adequate circulating blood volume is the most important requirement for a stable cardiovascular system during anaesthesia.

Liver disease

Drugs requiring metabolism by the liver should be used with caution. However, liver disease is rarely a major problem if kidney function is adequate.

Drug Interactions

Corticosteroids:
therapeutic doses of steroids depress the adrenal cortex. As a result the gland may be unable to secrete sufficient steroids in response to the stress of anaesthesia and surgery. Soluble steroids such as hydrocortisone or dexamethasone should be given intravenously during anaesthesia and surgery if the animal has recently been treated with steroids over a period of ten days or longer.

Insulin:
diabetics should be stabilised before anaesthesia. In this case anaesthesia should cause minimal disturbance if it is timed to interfere as little as possible with the patient's normal routine. A short period of hyperglycaemia is preferable to hypoglycaemia and 5% glucose may be infused if there is any likelihood of hypoglycaemia.

NSAIDs:
these drugs are usually highly protein bound and will displace the protein bound anaesthetics such as thiopentone. In theory this should result in increased sensitivity to the anaesthetic drug and smaller doses should be given.

Cardiac glycosides:
if an animal is well stabilised on cardiac glycosides it is probably better to continue treatment. However, these drugs may cause dysrhythmias and abnormal responses to anaesthetic drugs. If there is any likelihood of overdose, treatment should be stopped before anaesthesia.

Beta blockers:
these drugs alter the response of the cardiovascular system to anaesthetic drugs, in particular by preventing an increase in heart rate in response to hypotension. It may not be necessary to discontinue treatment but careful maintenance of a stable cardivascular system is essential.

Anticonvulsive therapy:
treatment should generally be continued but reduced doses of anaesthetics may be required.

Antibiotics:
aminoglycoside antibiotics (streptomycin, neomycin, gentamycin, etc.) may induce neuromuscular block resulting in respiratory insufficiency with some volatile agents (particularly ether).

Premedication:
the response of the animal to the drugs given as premedication gives a useful guide to its general health. Excessive depression resulting from small doses of sedatives suggests the need for caution and further investigation.

MONITORING

The aim of anaesthetic monitoring is to ensure the patient's well-being throughout anaesthesia. Continual assessment enables immediate remedial action to be taken if any problem arises. Measurements should be made regularly and frequently, (ie every 5—10 minutes) so that trends can be seen and any problems treated as soon as they arise. A written record is useful as it prompts regular measurement, shows up any trends and provides a useful record of all that has occurred should a problem arise, or if the animal has to be anaesthetised again.

The ABC must be maintained at all times.

Good monitoring forms the basis for maintenance of the ABC:

A = Airway.

A patent airway must be ensured at all times. An endotracheal tube does not guarantee a patent airway.

B = Breathing.

Adequate respiration is essential. General anaesthesia tends to depress respiration and if ventilation is inadequate IPPV must be supplied immediately, whatever the cause of the failure.

C = Circulation.

An adequate circulation must be maintained throughout anaesthesia. Circulatory function should be stabilised before surgery and blood and evaporative losses occurring during anaesthesia replaced immediately. Myocardial depression may be caused by anaesthetic overdose and should be treated as outlined in chapter 16.

WHAT TO MONITOR

Respiration

Respiratory pattern and rate should be monitored. Visual assessment of movement of the chest wall and of the rebreathing bag is necessary. Patency of the airway and respiratory function can be assessed. Respiratory effort that produces no movement of the rebreathing bag indicates that the airway is obstructed or that the endotracheal tube is not connected to the breathing circuit. Excessive respiratory effort that produces little, or delayed movement of the reservoir bag indicates an obstructed airway. Watching movement of the rebreathing bag is useful for subjective assessment of tidal volume, but detection of slight reduction in ventilation is not easy. A Wright's Respirometer can be used to measure tidal volume. However, these instruments increase dead space and the resistance to breathing and are not very robust. Respiration monitors with a detector placed in the airway which bleep as warm gas is expired are useful to indicate that the animal is breathing but do not indicate adequacy of ventilation.

Light anaesthesia, hypercapnia, painful stimulation and respiratory disease may result in rapid respiration. Anaesthetic overdose and fatigue decrease respiratory rate and depth. Shallow respiration, whether fast or slow, often results in inadequate ventilation.

Pulse

Pulse rate and quality should be assessed. Palpation of peripheral pulses using digital or lingual arteries is best as this gives the most information about circulation. Palpation of the femoral artery is also useful. Auscultation of heart beat tells less about the circulation but does demonstrate that the heart is still pumping. An oesophageal stethoscope is particularly useful for detection of the heart beat during head and neck surgery, in tiny patients or when the animal is covered in surgical drapes. Pulse monitors that produce a bleep triggered by the R wave of the ECG detect neither a pulse nor myocardial pumping action, but simply indicate that there is electrical activity in the heart. Such instruments are not recommended as they continue to bleep long after the myocardium has ceased to pump. Pulse oximeters and optical pulse detectors respond to changes in haemoglobin oxygen saturation or colour change, respectively, and are true peripheral pulse detectors. They are most effective used on the tongue, lip or toe web.

A strong peripheral pulse at a normal rate suggests that the circulation is adequate. However, hypercarbia results in bounding peripheral pulses so respiratory function must also be checked. Light anaesthesia, response to painful stimulation, hypovolaemia and anticholinergic agents, all increase heart rate. Myocardial depression from anaesthetic overdose and vagal stimulation may decrease heart rate. Both tachycardia and bradycardia may indicate that circulation is inadequate. Hypotension, hypovolaemia, myocardial depression and intense peripheral vasoconstriction result in a weak and thready pulse. This indicates inadequate circulation.

Mucous membranes

Colour and capillary refill time provide useful information. Assessment of colour is subjective but obvious changes can be detected. Capillary refill time (C.R.T.) is assessed by timing the return of colour to an area blanched by digital pressure. Approximately 2 seconds is normal.

Hypovolaemia, response to painful stimulation, peripheral vasoconstriction and anaemia result in pale mucous membranes. Hypoxaemia and cardiac failure result in cyanotic mucous membranes. Undetected failure of the oxygen supply while nitrous oxide is still being administered, results in navy blue mucous membranes. Slow C.R.T. indicates poor peripheral blood flow and may result from hypovolaemia and cardiovascular depression. A normal capillary refill time does not necessarily indicate that perfusion is adequate as normal refill times are seen when peripheral flow is sluggish due to cardiovascular failure and vasodilation.

Temperature

Core temperature is most effectively measured with a thermocouple placed in the oesophagus or pharynx. Rectal probes are less accurate, as rectal ballooning may occur. Clinical thermometers in the rectum can be used but have to be removed and shaken down between each reading. Palpation of extremities gives a useful subjective guide to peripheral temperature, although skin probe thermocouples are now commercially available and are more accurate.

General anaesthesia depresses normal temperature control mechanisms. Hypothermia is the most common consequence but hyperthermia occurs occasionally. Monitoring body temperature enables early treatment before severe changes occur. Temperature monitoring is especially important in the tiny patients which lose heat readily and in any prolonged surgery, particularly when large areas of wet tissue are exposed, as heat is lost in evaporation. Decreased peripheral temperature, particularly if the difference between core and periphery is widening, indicates poor peripheral circulation and is seen in shock.

Depth of anaesthesia

Depth of anaesthesia is assessed by taking into account clinical observation of the cardiovascular and respiratory systems, the response to surgical or other stimulus and the degree of muscular relaxation and eye position. Different anaesthetic agents have variable effects on these systems, so that only general rules can be applied. Monitors which measure the concentration of anaesthetic vapour in the breathing circuit can be used to maintain anaesthesia at a relatively constant depth by adjusting the anaesthetic supply to maintain a constant alveolar (end tidal) concentration. Approximately 1.5 MAC (minimum alveolar concentration that keeps 50% of patients anaesthetised during a standard stimulus) is usually required for most surgery. Additional intravenous or inhalational agents will reduce the MAC of the volatile agent.

In general, increases in respiratory and pulse rates, depth of respiration, muscle tone and response to stimuli indicate lightening anaesthesia. Decreases in these parameters indicate that anaesthesia is deepening. In many breeds of dog and cat, the eye rotates ventrally at a depth of anaesthesia suitable for most surgery. The eye is central during both light and very deep anaesthesia. These can usually be differentiated by lacrimation, which may be profuse in light anaesthesia but ceases as anaesthesia becomes very deep. All factors must be taken into account in assessing depth; reliance on one factor alone may be totally misleading.

Fluids

The nature and volume of fluids lost and supplied during anaesthesia and surgery should be recorded. Blood loss is estimated or measured as outlined in chapter 15. Urinary output is best measured (ml/hr) by inserting a urinary catheter and collecting the urine into a calibrated bag or bottle. Fluid input is monitored by regularly checking the infusion rate and assuring that the catheter has not become dislodged from the vein. Regular weighing of the infusion bag provides a more accurate estimate of how much fluid has been given. A set infusion rate is most easily maintained by using an infusion or syringe pump, but counting the drop rate is adequate if checked frequently. Measurement of total protein, haematocrit and central venous pressure may also be used in monitoring fluid balance during anaesthesia. These techniques are described in chapter 15.

Serious monitoring of fluid input and output is required primarily for major and prolonged surgery. However, assessment of any excessive losses, particularly of blood, should be performed in all cases. Continuous monitoring of fluid losses enables these to be replaced immediately, before the patient's condition deteriorates. Monitoring of input is equally important to ensure that the calculated replacement is actually taking place and to prevent overtransfusion. Simultaneous monitoring of the animal's cardiovascular system enables adjustment in fluid input to be made as necessary. Measurement of urinary output during surgery is a useful additional monitor of the cardiovascular system as normal urinary output will only occur if the kidneys are adequately perfused.

Electrocardiogram

Numerous ECG monitors are now available commercially; those made for human use are quite adequate. Output onto a screen, rather than paper, enables continuous assessment. Record is made using a minimum of three electrodes: one either side of the heart and one indifferent. During anaesthesia it is not essential to obtain standard lead recordings but simply to record a recognisable PQRST pattern to show changes in rhythm and configuration.

The ECG shows heart rate and electrical activity; it gives no information about the heart as a pump. Dysrhythmias and changes in the PQRST trace may be due to anaesthetic overdose, hypercarbia, hypoxia, acidosis and electrolyte imbalance. The general condition of the animal must be taken into account in order to ascertain the cause and to instigate any necessary treatment.

Arterial blood pressure

This is measured either directly, from an arterial catheter using an anaeroid manometer or electronic transducer, or indirectly, using a cuff and pulse detector. Doppler flow pulse detectors placed over the anterior metatarsal artery work well in the majority of dogs and cats.

Measurement of arterial blood pressure is not routinely carried out in small animal anaesthesia but provides useful direct information about the cardiovascular system that is particularly valuable for major surgery. Many anaesthetic agents are hypotensive, and hypotension is difficult to detect on clinical grounds alone. Accurate knowledge of arterial pressure enables remedial action to be taken before cardiovascular depression becomes severe and clinically obvious.

Blood gas, pH and electrolyte measurement

Arterial oxygen, carbon dioxide, pH, sodium and potassium, can be measured with sophisticated blood gas analysers and flame photometers. Although such facilities are rarely available in general practice, the information derived from such measurement is invaluable in assessing the well-being of the anaesthetised patient, since blood gas tensions and electrolytes are fundamental indicators of the state of body function.

Equipment

Normal function of all anaesthetic equipment should be ensured by regular, simple checks, both before and throughout anaesthesia. Correctly functioning equipment makes a substantial contribution to the well-being of the patient. These checks should include ensuring that gas flow and vaporizer setting remain as set, and particularly that the oxygen supply is adequate. Connector junctions, particularly in the breathing circuit, contents of vaporizer and the state of the soda lime, should also be regularly checked.

POST OPERATIVE CARE

Care of the patient during the recovery period is as important as that during anaesthesia. The animal should not be left unattended until it has recovered consciousness sufficiently for it, at least, to raise its head and preferably, to sit up.

Maintenance of the ABC is essential. The animal is particularly vulnerable to inadequate respiratory function and hypoxaemia in the recovery period. The CNS is still depressed and the animal less likely to be able to clear its airway if it becomes obstructed. In addition, the animal is now breathing air, 21% oxygen, after receiving supplementary oxygen during anaesthesia. Oxygen can be supplied by face mask or intranasal tube and, if voluntary respiration is inadequate, IPPV must be supplied until the animal is able to support itself. Fluid therapy should be continued in the recovery period if losses are still to be made up or maintenance requirements to be met.

Maintenance of normal temperature is important in the recovery period. A hypothermic animal metabolises most anaesthetic drugs very slowly, so recovery is prolonged. The condition thus tends to be self perpetuating. Insulation with blankets, plastic bubble packing or space blankets is effective. Heated pads are not very effective unless the animal is also insulated. A warm environment is important. Any fluids administered in this period should be heated to at least room temperature and preferably to 37° C.

Analgesia must be provided after any surgical procedure that is likely to result in post operative pain. It is most effective to give an analgesic parenterally before the animal regains consciousness and, in most cases, an opioid drug as described in chapter 9, will be required. Use of opioids in these circumstances may prolong the recovery period and carries the risk of respiratory depression. However, these are not major drawbacks as long as animals are not left to recover unattended.

General comfort must be attended to in the recovery period. Comfortable room temperature, suitable bedding, food, water and cleanliness go a long way to providing pleasant conditions for the patient. An empty bladder is essential for comfort and every dog should be carried or helped to a suitable place to urinate or have a urinary catheter in place if this is impossible. Cats should be given a litter tray. Human attention and a little TLC (tender loving care) is even more important.

FURTHER READING

HALL, L. W. and CLARKE, K. W. (1991). Veterinary Anaesthesia. Balliere Tindall. London.

HOULTON, J. E. F. and TAYLOR, P. M. (1987). Trauma management in the dog and cat. Wright. Bristol. 1-10, 101-116.

TAYLOR, P. M. and HOULTON, J. E. F. (1984). Post operative analgesia in the dog. A comparison of morphine, buprenorphine and pentazocine. J. Small Anim. Pract. **25** 437-451.

TAYLOR, P. M. (1988). Anaesthesia: established principles and new developments. In: Advances in Small Animal Practice. Ed: E. A. Chandler. Blackwell Scientific Publications. Oxford. 87-119.

CHAPTER 3

ANAESTHETIC EQUIPMENT AND SAFETY

R. S. Jones M.V.Sc., Dr. Med.Vet., D.V.Sc., D.V.A., F.I. Biol., F.R.C.V.S.

A number of machines are available for use in veterinary anaesthesia. The majority of them were designed for medical use, however, a limited number have been developed specifically for veterinary use in the U.K. Two publications have surveyed the available equipment (Hird, 1983)(Rex 1969).

Basic anaesthetic equipment consists of gas cylinders, reducing valves, pressure gauges, flowmeters and vaporisers (Figures 3.1 and 3.2).

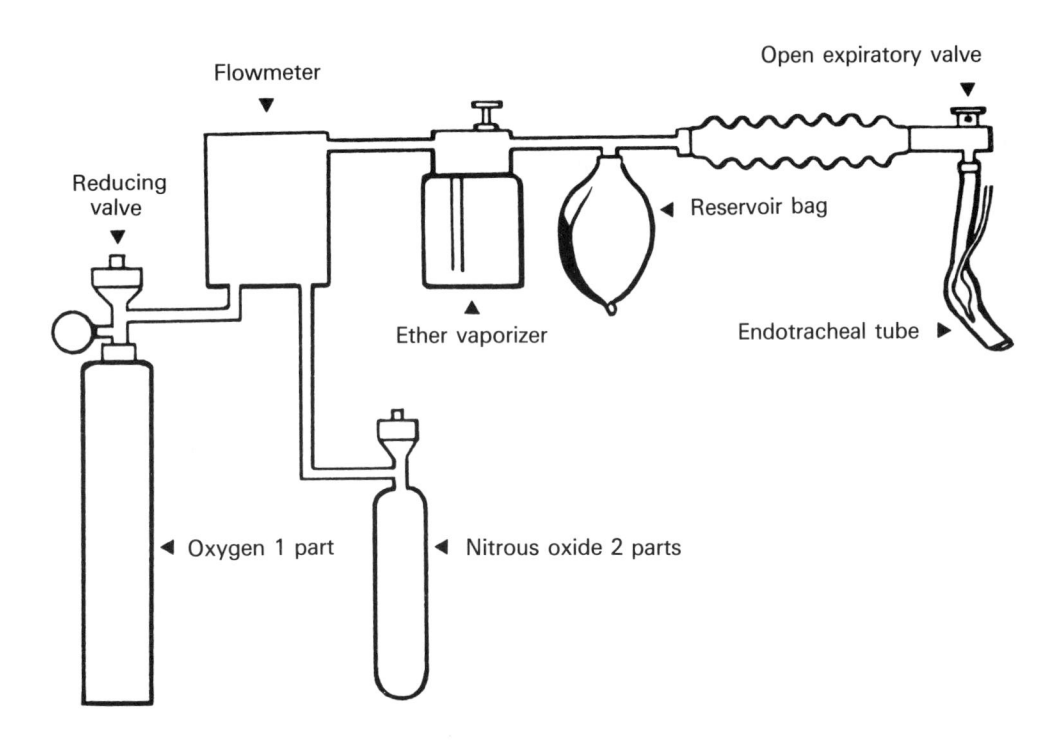

Figure 3.1

The apparatus for administering nitrous oxide/oxygen and a volatile agent in semi-closed circuit by endotracheal tube.

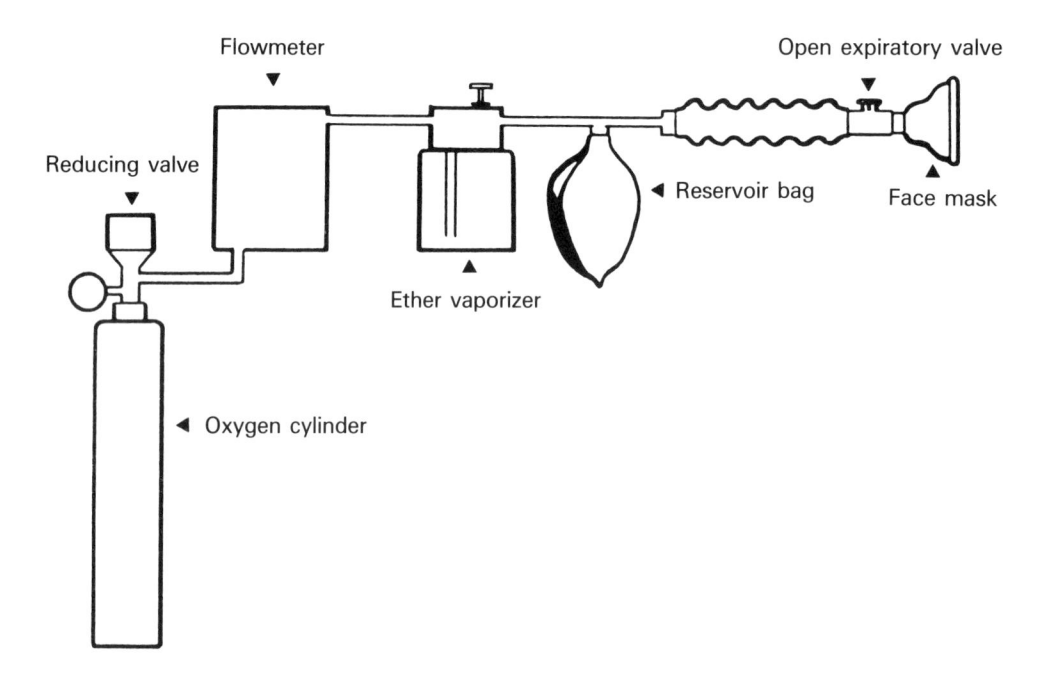

Figure 3.2
The apparatus for administering oxygen and ether in a semi closed circuit with a mask.

The Boyle's machine is the classic anaesthetic apparatus and there are a considerable number of variations on this machine. All are continuous flow machines with gases delivered from cylinders or pipelines by way of reducing valves to the flow meters, where the flow is controlled by a needle valve. One or more vaporisers are incorporated for use as required. The gases then pass to either a closed or semi-closed circuit.

1. **Trolley or Stand**

    a. Trolley Units have four wheels and one or two table surfaces as shelves on the machine. They usually incorporate a drawer and the more elaborate ones have a retractable writing surface. They have the advantage of a shelf (or shelves) on which can be placed an extra vaporiser, ventilator and/or monitoring equipment such as an ECG. They do, however, take up more space and need more cleaning and maintenance than stand units. They are, by necessity, much more expensive than stands.

        Manufacturers include:-

        Blease Medical   Blease Minor
        B. O. C. Medishield   Boyle Model M
        MIE Ltd.   Cavendish 250
        Penlon Ltd.   IM 500 Series

b. Stands have either three or four wheels in a tripod or cruciate arrangement. They have the advantage that they occupy less space than trolleys and are easier to clean. They are in general cheaper than trolleys, but have a variety of disadvantages, including the lack of provision for nitrous oxide. If the shelf is present at all, it is usually smaller than the trolley top.

Manufacturers include:-

B. O. C. Medishield	Boyle Petite and Boyle twin gas.
Bowring Engineering Ltd.	Tripod Stand — single or twin gas.
Alfred Cox (Surgical Ltd.)	Tripod Stand — single gas.
Vet. Equip. Co. Ltd.	Tripod Stand — twin gas.

2. Gas Cylinders

Gas cylinders are classified according to their size by letters from AA to J. They are made of molybdenum steel and are checked for defects by the manufacturers, from time to time, subjecting them to a number of tests. These include tensile strength, flattening impact and hydraulic tests.

Oxygen is supplied in cylinders coloured black with white necks, filled to a pressure of 132 atmospheres. The common sizes in use in veterinary anaesthesia are E (24 ft) and F (48 ft).

Nitrous oxide is supplied in blue-coloured cylinders, filled to a pressure of 51 atmospheres. Sizes D (200 gallons) and E (400 gallons) are commonly used. Cylinder outlet valves use the pin-index system, which makes it virtually impossible to connect the cylinders to an incorrect yoke.

3. Reducing Valves

Reducing valves are placed between the source of compressed gas (either cylinder or pipe-line) and the flowmeter. They allow delicate control of gas flows and continuous adjustments are not necessary to maintain a constant flow, despite any variations in pressure and temperature within the cylinders. The classic reducing valve is the Adams Valve which reduces the pressure to 40-75 k Pa. This has been superseded by the Medishield valves which operate by way of a toggle mechanism and reduce the pressure either to 810 k Pa (S valve), or to 450 k Pa (M valve).

4. Pressure Gauges

A pressure gauge may also be incorporated into the regulator. The pressure gauge indicates the quantity of gas within the cylinder.

5. Flowmeters

Flowmeters are required to control the flow of gas and also give an indication of the amount passing to the patient. They can be either of the variable or fixed orifice type. Whilst a large number of different types are available, the only one in common use is the Rotameter (a variable-orifice and fixed-pressure difference type). It is accurate with an error of $\pm 2\%$. In operation, the gas enters the bottom of a finely wrought glass tube which is slightly smaller in cross section at the bottom that at the top. The tubes, one for each gas, are enclosed in a glass cylinder. A metal float rides on the gas jet and the notches in its edge cause it to rotate. The height of the top of the metal float indicates the flow rate as the gas escapes between the rim of the float and the walls of the tube. The tubes must be vertical and the calibration is influenced both by the density and viscosity of each particular gas. A rotameter calibrated for one gas will not read true for another. Flow meters are calibrated for use at atmospheric pressure and hence they are inaccurate at high altitudes.

Occasional inaccuracies can occur if the float sticks in the tube due to static electricity, but this is only likely to be a problem at low flow rates. The float can occasionally jam at the top of the tube and the anaesthetist may then be unaware that the gas is flowing. This is more common with the small bobbins used for carbon dioxide, with very serious consequences.

6. Vaporisers

Vaporisers are employed when volatile liquids are used in anaesthesia. One or more vaporisers may be sited on a particular machine, depending on the personal choice of the veterinary surgeon and on economics. If more than one vaporiser is used, the liquid having the lowest boiling point should be vaporised first; thus the vapour from the first vaporiser is less likely to condense in the second vaporiser.

A wide variety of vaporisers are now available.

   a. **Boyle's Bottle**

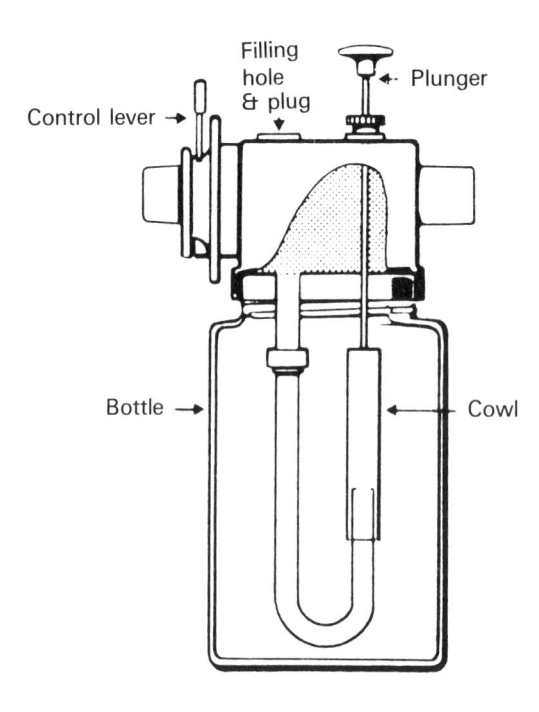

Figure 3.3
Boyle's bottle vaporiser.

One of the most commonly used vaporisers in veterinary anaesthesia is the Boyle's bottle (figure 3.3), which allows a fairly fine control of the concentration of the anaesthetic vapour by:-

i. Diverting a variable amount of gas from the flowmeters into the bottle by the ON-OFF switch. When the lever is 'off', none of the gas enters the bottle and conversely, when it is 'on', all the gas enters the bottle.

ii. Passing the gases through a J-shaped tube before they enter the bottle. The end of the J-shaped tube, through which the gases emerge, is covered by a hood which can be moved up and down by moving the metal rod attached to it which protrudes through the top of the vaporiser. The nearer the hood is to the surface, the nearer the gases are deflected to it (in the ether and trichlorethylene bottles, the gases can be diverted under the surface of the liquid and bubble through it, but not in the halothane bottle).

One disadvantage of the Boyle's bottle, is that, as the gas picks up the vapour and flows from the bottle, further vaporisation occurs. This continuous process is accompanied by a fall in temperature of the liquid and hence a corresponding fall in the speed of vaporisation. If there is a constant flow, the temperature continues to fall and consequently the concentration of vapour delivered also falls, until the loss of heat by evaporation is balanced by the flow of heat from the exterior. A number of methods have been used to overcome this problem. Water baths have been placed around the vaporiser to prevent heat loss, but are not very efficient. Bimetallic bars have been used to give a variation in the inlet port of the vaporiser with temperature. An apparatus has also been designed to provide a saturated vapour which can be diluted to obtain the required concentration.

b. 'Tec' Vaporisers.

The commonest vaporisers using one of these principles are of the 'tec' type. They are available for most volatile anaesthetic agents but only the 'Fluotec' (halothane) and 'Pentec' (methoxyflurane) are in common use in veterinary anaesthesia. This type of vaporiser utilises the principle of a bimetallic strip as a temperature compensator. The gas, on entering the vaporiser, splits into two streams, one of which by-passes, while the other enters the vaporising chamber where it becomes saturated with vapour. The concentration of the vapour leaving the vaporiser can be calculated if the saturated vapour pressure of the anaesthetic agent and the splitting ratio of the two streams are known. The 'Tec' vaporiser remains accurate with changes in temperature, passage of time, variation of the amount of liquid and the gas flow. A number of 'Fluotec' models are available:

>Mark II, 4% and 10%
>
>Mark III, 5% and 8% (veterinary model)

The MK III gives a high output at low flow rates and is linear at all flows. A MKII model 'Pentec', is available with an output of up to 1.5 %. Mark IV models are now available.

c. Other Vaporisers

i.   The Goldman vaporiser is a simple apparatus without temperature compensation and is rarely used in veterinary anaesthesia, except possibly in-circuit, due to its low output.

ii. The Copper Kettle vaporiser is constructed of copper, which allows heat to pass rapidly from the room to the liquid. It is very efficient and uses the principle of metering the variable flow of carrier gas (oxygen to nitrous oxide-oxygen) through the volatile liquid and mixing the saturated vapour with known volumes of diluent gas, to provide an accurate control over the final vapour concentration.

iii. The Drager vaporiser is a very accurate vaporiser which is similar to the Copper Kettle.

iv. A number of other manufacturers produce vaporisers for volatile agents but they are all used to a limited extent in veterinary anaesthesia.

d. Position of Vaporiser in the Circuit

When circle systems are used for inhalational anaesthesia, the vaporiser may be either inside or outside the circuit. It is not possible to place the vaporiser inside with a to-and-fro system. The system of vaporiser inside the circuit is only commonly used with halothane.

With the vaporiser inside the circuit (VIC), a relatively inefficient vaporiser such as a Goldman is used. The halothane is vaporised by the patient's respiratory effort, hence the deeper the breathing the more halothane is vaporised. Respiration becomes depressed as anaesthesia deepens and less halothane is vaporised, which acts as a built in safety mechanism. It is a very economical system when it is used in closed circuit with a basal oxygen flow. Controlled respiration must be used carefully as it can release a large amount of halothane vapour into the circle system.

With the vaporiser outside the circuit (VOC), the volatile agent is vaporised by the flow of fresh gases and hence nitrous oxide can be used. If the flow is small, then the vaporiser must be efficient at, and calibrated for, low flows. Known concentrations can be delivered to the circuit and inspired concentrations estimated.

7. Warning Devices and Safety Checks.

It may be considered desirable to fit a warning device to an anaesthetic machine to indicate that the oxygen supply is failing. Ideally, it should emit an audible and visual signal and not depend on another gas pressure to provide the warning. The 'Bosun' device relies on nitrous oxide for its audible signal and hence is not ideal. Newer devices are now available which depend solely on the failing oxygen pressure.

Safety checks of anaesthetic apparatus are essential to prevent accidents from cross-connections. A technique has been described by Adams and Henville (1979). Initially, the apparatus should be disconnected from all piped gases and the cylinders turned off.

Then:
1. Check that full cylinders are properly attached to their yokes and are turned off.
2. Open the O_2 and N_2O flow-meter valves 2 to 3 full turns and ensure that the others are closed. No flow occurs.
3. Turn on O_2 cylinder. Check O_2 gauge for contents. O_2 flow-meter should register a flow — adjust to test flow 4 litres/min. If any N_2O flow registers, reject machine.
4. Turn on N_2O cylinder and check that N_2O meter registers a flow. If O_2 flow changes, reject machine.
5. Set the O_2 failure device in operation if not automatic.
6. Turn off O_2 cylinder. Check that O_2 bobbin falls completely to bottom of tube. Check that O_2 failure device works. If O_2 flow meter registers any flow when N_2O only turned on, reject machine.
7. Complete check by occluding machine outlet and ensure that pressure relief valve on back bar is operative (where fitted).

Circle systems should be checked for leaks by occluding the patient outlet, closing the overflow valve and filling the system with oxygen and determining whether the pressure in the system is maintained. If there are leaks, they should be detected and remedied. Non-rebreathing or semi-closed systems should be checked in a similar manner.

8. Face Masks

Face masks are available in malleable latex rubber for use in cats and dogs. Despite the wide variations in the configuration and size of the face of domestic animals, these masks can be moulded around their contours. They are held in position either by a harness or elastoplast and produce a reasonably tight seal. Four sizes of the Hall masks are available.

9. Laryngoscopes

A large number of different types of laryngoscopes have been developed as an essential aid to endotracheal intubation in the human subject. Whilst they are not essential in domestic animals, they can be valuable under certain conditions; such as in small dogs and cats and in animals with oral or pharyngeal pathology. A laryngoscope consists of a handle, which holds a battery, and a detachable blade. The detachable blades vary in size and shape. The common ones are either of the straight or Magill type, or of the curved or McIntosh type. The Magill type is preferable for use in animals and one each of the standard infant, child and adult blades are recommended. The blades are detachable for sterilisation by boiling or autoclaving.

10. Endotracheal Tubes.

Intubation of the trachea was practised experimentally in animals a number of centuries ago. It is, however, only in this century, that the technique has been employed routinely in human anaesthesia and only in the last quarter of a century in animals. Those in common use are the Magill mineralised rubber tubes, although polythene (polyvinyl chloride) ones are now available. The number of the tube corresponds to its internal diameter in millimeters. In animals, the thicker walled, oral, red rubber tubes are preferred. Tubes with an internal diameter of greater than 5 millimeters are supplied with inflatable cuffs. These are used to ensure an airtight seal between the tube and the trachea. The pilot balloon indicates the state of the cuff in the trachea. Cuffs should not be inflated to a greater pressure that that needed to prevent audible leakage of gas on compression of the reservoir bag. Tubes should be washed with soapy water both inside and outside. In order to prevent irritation to the trachea all tubes should be washed thoroughly in clean water to remove all traces of detergent or soap. Autoclaving is the best way of sterilising them, but tends to shorten their life.

The techniques of endotracheal intubation in the dog and cat will be familiar to most veterinary surgeons:

i. **Endotracheal Intubation in the Dog.**

This is a relatively simple procedure. Once anaesthesia has been induced, a gag is placed between the canine teeth and the head is held up by an assistant. The tongue is pulled forwards out of the mouth with the left hand. The lubricated tube is placed in the right hand and its tip is used to elevate the soft palate and depress the epiglottis. The arytenoids are then visible and the tube is passed between them. The tube should be inserted so that its cuffed area lies in the cervical trachea between the larynx and the first rib. The cuff should then be inflated to provide an air tight seal.

ii. **Endotracheal Intubation in the Cat.**

The larynx of the cat is very susceptible to spasm (Rex, 1970). The difficulty can be overcome by a number of techniques or a combination of them. Deep anaesthesia can be induced and the tube introduced into the larynx. Alternatively, the larynx of the cat can be sprayed with a local anaesthetic solution once anaesthesia has been induced. Care should be taken not to administer a large volume of local anaesthetic (one or two sprays is sufficient) or else signs of toxicity (convulsions, respiratory arrest) may be produced. Another method is to administer 1-2 mg of suxamethonium to the cat by the intravenous route and, once the animal is paralysed, pass the tube into the larynx. The actual technique is very similar to that employed in the dog, although in view of the cat's small size, a laryngoscope can be valuable. A stilette may also be helpful to stiffen flexible, small endotracheal tubes.

11. Ventilators

A full discussion of the many ventilators available is to be found in the book by Mushin *et al.* (1969). A number of methods have been used for classifying ventilators but basically they are of two types:

a. **Pressure Preset** — in which pressure builds up to a preset level irrespective of the volume delivered.

b. **Volume Preset** — which delivers a set volume of gas. Pressure will rise to overcome any obstruction, but a safety blow-off is normally incorporated at about 30cm. H_2O.

Mode of Action.

An understanding of the mechanism of the cycling of ventilators is important for the effective use of the machines. Cycling, basically refers to the mechanism which brings about the change from the inspiratory to the expiratory phase. Ventilators are either pressure, volume or time cycled.

A knowledge of the wave forms produced by ventilators is essential. They can either be pressure or flow generators. In pressure-generator ventilators a rapid inflationary stroke produces a square wave form and prolongation of the inspiratory phase does not increase filling of the lungs. Flow-generators produce a triangular wave form as the inflation pressure rises steadily throughout the inspiratory phase.

Ventilators can be driven either by electricity or gas pressure. Electrically driven machines are in common use but there is a risk of explosions if inflammable anaesthetic gases or vapours are used. Compressed gas can be obtained either from cylinders or a pipe line. An alternative source of compressed gas is a compressor. Some of the ventilators which have been used in veterinary anaesthesia are:

i. **Radcliffe.**

A pressure preset and time cycled machine which is electrically driven. A reservoir bag is raised by an arm and compressed by adjustable weights. A negative phase and closed circuit system are incorporated.

ii. **Bird.**

Developed and used widely in the United States, the Bird is a flow generator which is time and pressure cycled. A number of different models are available with different capacities. An anaesthetic attachment, which consists basically of a 'bag in bottle', is available.

iii. **Manley.**

A minute volume divider which is operated by the flow of gas delivered from an anaesthetic machine. Once the tidal volume has been set the ventilator delivers the minute volume from the anaesthetic machine at the appropriate rate.

iv. **Miniature Ventilators.**

A number, all having similar features, have been described by Hall and Massey (1969). They are all small, inexpensive and simple. They will fit on any anaesthetic machine which delivers a flow of gas. The elasticity of a distended reservoir bag is used to provide the driving force for inspiration and once the pressure in the bag rises it releases a bobbin, which is held by a magnet, allowing inspiration to take place. These are also minute volume dividers.

12. Scavenging Systems.

In order to collect the waste gases from anaesthetic systems, a system of collecting valve and tubing is required to duct the effluent to the atmosphere. They can be classified as either passive or active systems. In a passive system, the total flow resistance should not exceed 50 k Pa at 30 litres per minute and copper pipes of 35 mm outer diameter are satisfactory. A T-termination with a downward right angle bend at each end is to be preferred. An assisted passive system can be used by employing a theatre ventilating system which must be of the non recirculating type. With an active system, the patient should be protected from a negative pressure greater than 100 Pa. There should be a reservoir bag in order to protect the patient from subatmospheric pressure. The Cardiff Aldosorber has been used to remove anaesthetic vapours by activated charcoal. It does **not** remove nitrous oxide.

13. Care and Maintenance of Anaesthetic Machines.

Most anaesthetic machines require little in the way of general maintenance. Where maintenance contracts are available, it is best to have the units checked and serviced at least once a year. Particular attention should be paid to precision vaporisers; in the case of halothane they may stick due to the thymol present in the preparation. They are best serviced by the manufacturer. It is difficult to be precise on the time intervals as this will depend a great deal on the amount of usage.

14. Maintenance of other Anaesthetic Equipment.

After use, all the rubber equipment (tubing, bags, tubes and masks), should be washed thoroughly with an antiseptic soap and allowed to drain. Care should be taken to rinse any disinfectant off the rubber thoroughly. The absorber should be protected from the air and, once the soda lime is exhausted, it should be emptied and the canister washed and carefully dried before re-charging. All vaporisers, flowmeters and cylinder valves should be turned off after use and, unless they are in daily use, all vaporisers should be emptied of volatile anaesthetic agents. Any valves in the circuits (not machine) which tend to stick, should be dismantled and cleaned and dried thoroughly. Any rubber equipment which shows signs of wear should be replaced immediately, both on the grounds of efficiency and of safety. In summary, anaesthetic equipment is a precision instrument and should be treated as such.

REFERENCES

ADAMS, A. P. and HENVILLE, J. D. (1979) in *Recent Advances in Anaesthesia and Analgesia.* 13th Ed. Hewer, C. L. and Atkinson, R. S. Churchill Livingstone, Edinburgh.

HALL, L. W. and MASSEY, G. M. (1969). Three miniature lung ventilators. *Vet. Rec.* **85**, 432.

HIRD, J. F. R. (1982). *Anaesthetic equipment in Manual of Practice Improvement.* BSAVA Publications.

HIRD, J. F. R. and CARLUCCI, F. (1978). A new anaesthetic circuit for use in the dog. *J. small Anim. Pract.* **19**, 277.

MUSHIN, W. W., RENDELL-BAKER, L., THOMPSON, P. W. and MAPLESON, W. W. (1980). *Automatic Ventilation of the Lungs.* 3rd Ed. Blackwell.

REX, M. A. E. (1969). Anaesthetic machine survey. *N. Z. vet. J.* **17**, 113.

REX, M. A. E. (1970). A review of the structural and functional basis of laryngospasm and a discussion of the nerve pathways involved in the reflex and its clinical significance in man and animals. *Brit. J. Anaesth.* **42**, 891.

FURTHER READING

HALL, L. W. and CLARKE, K. W. (1991). *Veterinary Anaesthesia.* 9th ed. Balliere Tindall.

LUMB, W. V. and JONES, E. W. (1984). *Veterinary Anaesthesia. 2nd ed.* Lea and Febiger, Philadelphia.

SHORT, C. E. (1987). *Principles and Practice of Veterinary Anaesthesia.* Williams and Wilkins, Baltimore.

CHAPTER 4

ANALGESIA

A. M. Nolan M.V.B., D.V.A., M.R.C.V.S.

INTRODUCTION

It is the duty of the veterinary surgeon to prevent or alleviate pain in animals.

Assessment of pain in animals is fraught with difficulties of interpretation. Anthropomorphism based on human experiences may not be appropriate as emotional and psychological factors influence the human reaction to pain. However, as all mammals have the same basic physiological structure, it is reasonable to assume that what is painful to man is likely to be painful in animals. A lack of ability on the part of the observer to identify a dog or cat's behaviour pattern as indicative of a response to pain, does not negate the existence of pain.

Recognition of Pain

Acute severe pain. Vocalisation and guarding behaviour either spontaneous or evoked if the animal is moved or touched. Aggressive behaviour and self mutilation may also indicate severe pain.

Chronic pain. Skeletal pain may be detected by the pressure of lameness, stiffness or difficulty in standing or sitting. Pain associated with chronic abdominal, aural or other organ pathologies, is more difficult to assess. Mild deviations from normal behaviour patterns; for example, decrease in appetite or reduced interspecies interaction, may be apparent only to the owners.

USE OF ANALGESICS

1. Control of acute pain. Perhaps the most common indication for the use of analgesic agents is the treatment of post-surgical pain. They are also of use in acute medical cases.
2. Control of chronic pain such as skeletal pain.
3. During anaesthesia. Analgesic agents may be used as part of a balanced anaesthetic technique, thus decreasing the amount of inhalation or intravenous (I/V) anaesthetic agent required.
4. In a neuroleptanalgesic mixture — to provide sedation and facilitate handling of fractious animals.

ANALGESIC DRUGS AVAILABLE

1. Opioids
2. Non-steroidal anti-inflammatory drugs (NSAIDSs). Used in the treatment of mild and low grade chronic pain.
3. Local anaesthetic drugs.
4. Miscellaneous drugs: e.g. ketamine, xylazine, medetomidine.

OPIOIDS

The opioid drugs are all chemically related and have been developed in an attempt to produce a safe, effective analgesic.

They may be classified into three groups with a range of activity from pure agonists (e.g. morphine) to partial agonists (e.g. buprenorphine) to pure antagonists (e.g. naloxone).

They should be used in the treatment of severe pain such as that arising from surgery or trauma.

Legal requirements

Many of the opioid drugs are classified as controlled drugs (C.D.) under Schedules 2 and 3 of the Misuse of Drugs Act 1971. These drugs are subject to strict regulations concerning their purchase, use and safekeeping. Stringent recording of their use in every animal is essential.

The RCVS publication 'Legislation affecting the veterinary profession in Great Britain' (1978) provides full details on the regulations governing the purchase and use of controlled drugs and veterinary surgeons should familiarise themselves with these controls. However, many of the newer partial agonists, e.g. buprenorphine, are free from the stringent controls of the Misuse of Drugs Act, (1971), due to their lack of ability to induce an addictive response in man.

General Effects of the Opioid Analgesics

The opioid analgesics produce a wide range of effects, which may be modified depending on the species, the choice of drug, the dose, the presence or absence of pain and the concurrent administration of other drugs. The major effects are summarised below:

- a. Analgesia
- b. Respiratory depression
- c. Sedation or excitement
- d. Nausea, vomiting, defaecation
- e. Depression of cough reflex
- f. Tolerance and dependence (only on prolonged administration)

The opioid analgesics are used mainly to provide analgesia or as part of a neuroleptanalgesic mixture, and as such the other effects may be considered in the whole as unwanted side effects.

Respiratory depression is potentially one of the most serious side effects of the opioid analgesics. However, it is rarely a problem in dogs and cats, and should not be considered as a contra-indication to the routine uses of opioids in clinical practice. If respiratory depression is encountered, a narcotic antagonist may be used (although this will, in addition, reverse the analgesic effects), or if occurring during general anaesthesia, ventilation may be carried out and the depth of anaesthesia lightened. The partial agonists have an upper limit to the severity of respiratory depression produced.

OPIOID AGONISTS

1. **Morphine** (C.D.)

    Morphine is a potent, reliable analgesic for use in the treatment of severe pain in dogs and cats.

    ### Use in dogs.

    Morphine causes analgesia and mild sedation in the dog and is used for both analgesia when required, and for premedication. Recommended dose rates are 0.1–0.25mg/kg given intramuscularly, to induce reliable analgesia. The duration of action is around 4–5 hours. Side effects include vomiting, although this is less likely in the animal in pain, and respiratory depression. Gastrointestinal effects are complex and result in initial stimulation (vomiting, defaecation) followed by a decrease in gut motility. Morphine is contraindicated in the treatment of pain associated with acute pancreatitis or biliary obstruction due to the spasm produced in gut sphincters and should be used with care in the animal with head injuries as it increases intracranial pressure. Cardiovascular effects at the recommended dose rates are minimal.

    ### Use in cats

    Morphine (0.1–0.2 mg/kg I/M, S/C) has a longer duration of action in the cat (6–8 hours) than in the dog. Excitement may occur at high doses.

2. **Papaveretum,** 'Omnopon', (Roche, C.D.)

    Papaveretum is a mixture of opium alkaloids containing 50% morphine. Its effects are similar to morphine when used at twice the dose rate (0.2—0.4 mg/kg, I/M).

3. **Pethidine** (C.D.)

    Pethidine is a synthetic opioid widely used for analgesia and premedication. It is considerably less potent than morphine and has a shorter duration of action but a more rapid onset of effect. Pethidine does not induce vomiting or defaecation and its atropine-like spasmolytic activity may make it a useful agent in the treatment of abdominal pain.

    ### Use in Dogs

    Dose rates of 3—4 mg/kg given intramuscularly produce reliable analgesia lasting 2.5—3.5 hours. Old animals and those with hepatic disease, require smaller doses to provide analgesia (1—2 mg/kg, I/M). Large doses (5 mg/kg) injected rapidly I/V may cause profound hypotension due to histamine release. Respiratory depression is of othe same order as that produced with any opioid drug when used at clinically effective doses.

    ### Use in Cats

    Dose rates of 5 mg/kg I/M produce short lasting, effective analgesia (2 hours).

4. **Methadone,** 'Physeptone', (Wellcome C.D.)

    Methadone produces good analgesia in the dog although the sedative effects are less than seen with morphine. Dose rates between 0.1—0.2 mg/kg, produce analgesia lasting approximately 4 hours.

5. **Fentanyl,** 'Sublimaze', (Janssen Pharmaceutical C.D.)

    Fentanyl is a potent analgesic with a rapid onset (1 minute) and a short duration of action (20—30 minutes). It is used mainly to provide analgesia during surgery when given intravenously (2—5 μg/kg). It may also be used in the initial post operative period to control severe pain or in combination with a sedative/tranquilliser as part of a neuroleptanalgesic technique. Fentanyl produces bradycardia when injected I/V which may be reversed with atropine. Respiratory depression may be a problem in the anaesthetised dog, necessitating artificial ventilation for a short period. In the conscious dog, panting may be seen.

Partial Agonist Opioid Analgesics

The partial agonists are drugs which can antagonise (to varying degrees) the actions of morphine, pethidine, fentanyl and others, but which themselves have sufficient agonist activity to be used in their own right.

Advantages: Not subjected to controlled drugs regulations (except pentazocine); vomiting seldom occurs.

Disadvantages: Analgesia may not be as intense; variable responses.

1. **Pentazocine** 'Fortral',(Winthrop C.D.)

    Pentazocine provides good post-operative analgesia and sedation when administered at dose rates of 2 mg/kg I/M. The duration of clinical analgesia can vary from 2—3 hours although sedation may be present for longer. It is equally effective in dogs and cats. It is also available in tablet form for oral use.

2. **Buprenorphine** 'Temgesic',(Reckitt & Colman)

    Buprenorphine is a potent analgesic used in dogs and cats. It has a slow onset of action (30—45 minutes) after I/M or I/V injection and therefore must be given well in advance of the end of surgery if used to provide post-operative analgesia. The quality and duration of analgesia may be variable, but on average, clinical analgesia lasts about 4 hours. Sedation is also a feature of the drugs effect and it is a useful component of neuroleptanalgesic mixtures. Doses of 4—10 μg/kg I/M are used in the dog and cat. Higher doses may result in less analgesia. The effects of buprenorphine are difficult to reverse with opioid antagonists, hence, if respiratory depression should occur (this is rarely seen), doxapram can be used to stimulate respiration.

3. **Butorphanol** 'Torbugesic', (C-Vet)

    Butorphanol has good sedative properties and may be used combined with a sedative in neuroleptanalgesic mixtures. Its analgesic effects are variable. Doses of 0.5 mg/kg I/M produce analgesia of approximately 3 hours duration in dogs, while in cats, effective analgesic doses may vary from 0.2–0.8 mg/kg.

4. **Nalbuphine** 'Nubain', (Dupont)

    Nalbuphine is an analgesic which has been little used in this country. Like butorphanol, its effects appear somewhat variable. Doses of 0.5 mg/kg I/M are recommended for use in the dog, but it offers no advantage over any other available analgesics. Its use in the cat is not recommended.

Opioid Antagonists

Pure antagonists, such as naloxone, have no activity when used alone, but will antagonise the effects of drugs with agonist activity.

Naloxone 'Narcan', (Winthrop)

Reasons for Use:

1. To reverse any undesirable effects of the opioid agonists. However, in addition to antagonising respiratory depression, analgesia will also be reversed.

2. To counteract the effects of accidental injection of potent opioid drugs into operating theatre personnel.

Problems of Use:

1. Attention must be paid to the relative duration of action of the agonist vs antagonist. Naloxone has a short duration of action (approx. 30 minutes), and an animal may relapse after the effects have waned.

2. If naloxone is used to reverse respiratory depression, no analgesia can be provided for the dog or cat as further opioid analgesics will be ineffective until the naloxone has been metabolised.

Recommended dose rates 0.02–0.04 mg/kg I/V or to effect. Repeat if necessary after 3–5 minutes.

Diprenorphine 'Small Animal Revivon', (C-Vet)

Although commonly classified as an antagonist, diprenorphine does have some weak analgesic activity when injected alone. It is marketed as a specific antagonist to the potent opioid etorphine and its usefulness is limited.

NSAIDs

These drugs are ineffective in controlling such severe pain as commonly occurs after surgery, but are useful in treating chronic pain associated with orthopaedic or other disease problems, or in the days following surgery. Many of these drugs are very toxic in both the dog and cat and care must be taken with dosage, frequency of dosing and monitoring for possible side effects. Extrapolation of doses from the human literature is unwise.

NSAIDs in dog and cat

DRUG	ROUTE	DOG	CAT
Phenylbutazone	Oral	10-20 mg/kg daily	10 mg/kg daily
Aspirin	Oral	25 mg/kg t.i.d.	25 mg/kg 48 hourly
Mefenamic Acid (Ponstan: Parke-Davis)	Oral	10 mg/kg b.i.d.	
Flunixin	Oral I/V	1 mg/kg daily	
Piroxicam	Oral	0.3 mg/kg 48 hourly	

LOCAL ANAESTHETIC DRUGS

By definition, these drugs provide analgesia. Their use in the treatment of pain, however, is limited to their own use peri-operatively, generally following thoracic surgery. Bupivicaine 'Marcain' (duration of action up to 6 hours), infiltrated around the intercostal nerves, can result in profound analgesia.

MISCELLANEOUS DRUGS

Ketamine 'Vetalar', (Parke-Davis)

Ketamine has not been used as an analgesic drug in animals although it does possess analgesic properties when used in subanaesthetic doses and has been used in man to control post-operative pain.

Recommended dose rates for use in cats; 1-2 mg/kg I/M or S/C.

Methoxyflurane 'Metofane', (C-Vet Ltd)

Methoxyflurane is a volatile anaesthetic agent with good analgesic properties (see Chapter 8). Elimination of methoxyflurane from the body is slow, thus resulting in effective analgesia.

Nitrous Oxide (N_2O)

N_2O is a good analgesic agent and may be administered for short periods of time with oxygen (66% N_2O, 34% O_2 to provide analgesia. However, the analgesic effect only persists as long as the N_2O is administered.

Xylazine 'Rompun', (Bayer) Medetomidine

These drugs, although not used widely in dogs and cats as such, have good analgesic properties. Low doses of xylazine may be useful in controlling pain of visceral origin (0.2-0.4 mg/kg I/M), in both dogs and cats. The profound side effects (sedation, hypotension, bradycardia) preclude its use at higher doses.

Recommendation for the Use of Analgesics

1. Following trauma.

    Opioids are recommended for the acute pain likely to arise following trauma. Avoid morphine if the animal has head injuries.

2. Pre-operatively.

    Opioids, given either alone or in conjunction with a sedative, will alleviate pain prior to surgery, enhance sedation and decrease the amount of anaesthetic required during surgery.

3. Post-operatively.

    Opioid analgesics are the drugs of choice in the immediate post-operative period, for the severe pain caused by, e.g., thoracic, orthopaedic, aural and abdominal surgery. Morphine or pethidine will provide effective, predictable analgesia.

    Note: all analgesics are most effective when given before pain is experienced, i.e. before the animal regains consciousness.

4. Chronic pain.

    NSAIDs most commonly used; e.g. mefenamic acid. Care must be taken with dosage to avoid toxic side effects. Pentazocine tablets may be used to treat severe pain.

5. Nursing care.

    Minimisation of discomfort by attention to the animal's general well-being through good nursing care will enhance the quality of pain relief by an analgesic drug. A dry, warm bed, support for a fractured limb, an empty bladder and human contact, will help to reduce the distress associated with painful conditions.

FURTHER READING

HALL, L. W, and CLARKE, K. W. (1991). *Veterinary Anaesthesia* 9th ed. Balliere Tindall.
Legislation affecting the veterinary profession in Great Britain (1978) Chapter III, Royal College of Veterinary Surgeons.
TAYLOR, P. M. (1985). *Analgesia in the dog and cat.* In 'Practice', **7,** 5—13.
WATERMAN, A. E. (1988). *Analgesia in Dogs and Cats.* In 'Advances in Small Animal Medicine'. Balliere Tindall.

CHAPTER 5

PREMEDICATION AND SEDATION

K. W. Clarke M.A., Vet. MB., D. Vet Med., D.V.A., M.R.C.V.S.

PREMEDICATION

Premedication prior to general anaesthesia is an integral part of the anaesthetic technique employed. The premedicant used affects the whole further course of events and the doses of general anaesthetic agents given must be modified accordingly.

The aims of premedication are as follows:

To calm and control the patient. This facilitates smooth induction, increases safety as fear may cause a dangerous level of adrenaline release and makes the process more pleasant for patient and anaesthetist.

To relieve pre-operative pain. Where this exists, the patient will not become calm without the administration of an analgesic. Such analgesics also continue to exert an effect throughout surgery and even in the post-operative period.

To reduce the total dose of anaesthetic.

To reduce unwanted autonomic side effects. These include the parasympathetic effects of excessive salivation and bronchial secretions and of bradycardia through increased vagal tone as well as adrenaline induced cardiac arrhythmias.

To reduce other unwanted side effects such as nausea, vomiting and post-operative excitement.

The drugs and doses chosen will depend on

1. The apparent age, condition and temperament of the animal.
2. The presence or absence of pain.
3. The anaesthetic technique to follow.
4. Any anticipated complications.
5. Post-operative requirements.
6. Other considerations, e.g. the foetus at caesarian section.

DRUGS EMPLOYED FOR PREMEDICATION

Premedication is usually carried out using one or more of the following drugs.

Sedative type drugs.

These are used to calm the patient, improving induction and recovery and reducing the quantities of anaesthetics used. Such drugs are an integral part of the anaesthetic technique, and the subsequent dose of anaesthetic drugs required and the duration of anaesthia, are dependent on the dose and type of sedative employed. Whether to employ light or heavy sedative premedication is the choice of the anaesthetist, but it is essential to understand the possible drug interactions as overdose of anaesthetic drugs subsequent to heavy premedication, is one of the commonest causes of anaesthetic emergencies. It is also important to allow adequate time for the sedative drugs used to exert their full effect before anaesthesia is induced, so that the required dose of induction agent can be correctly assessed.

The sedative drugs which may be employed for premedication are discussed in the subsequent section.

Analgesics.

When opioid drugs (chapter 4) are employed as premedicant agents, they may contribute to pre-operative, peri-operative and post-operative analgesia, depending on the duration of action and potency of the opioid selected. Their effects may be synergistic with both sedatives and anaesthetic drugs used and respiratory depression may be enhanced. Any remaining effects from opioids administered pre-operatively must also be considered when choosing post-operative analgesics.

Parasympathetic antagonists.

These are included in premedication to reduce salivation and prevent bradycardia. They are essential if drugs, such as ether, which cause excessive salivation, are used and are important where surgery is likely to stimulate vagally induced reflexes (e.g. surgery of the eye, ears, larynx etc.). They are also needed in some techniques employing neuromuscular blocking agents (chapter 9). The necessity for their routine use in the dog is controversial, but most authorities agree that they should be used routinely in the cat as in this species even normal salivation can result in respiratory obstruction.

The use of parasympathetic antagonists is contra-indicated in the presence of a pre-existing tachycardia.

Drugs used as parasympathetic antagonists include:-

Atropine. atropine sulphate, 0.5 mg/ml.
Many preparations available. Dose rates are not critical in either cats or dogs and those commonly used range from 0.02-0.1 milligrams (mg) /kg (i.e. from 0.25 mls of 0.5 mg/ml solution for a kitten or toy dog to 2 mls for a large dog) and can be given by the intramuscular (I/M), subcutaneous (S/C), or intravenous (I/V), routes.

Side effects: the pupil is widely dilated, particularly in cats. Initial slowing of the heart may occur through a central stimulating action on the vagus, before the blocking action results in tachycardia. Gross overdose results in central stimulation with convulsions.

Contra-indications: pre-existing tachycardia.

Glycopyrrolate. 'Robinul', (Robins).
This drug has recently been introduced in medical and veterinary anaesthesia. It is claimed that it has less central and occular effects than has atropine. Also, it does not cause as much tachycardia, but still prevents vagally induced bradycardia. Doses of 0.01 mg/kg have been used for premedication in cats and dogs.

Hyoscine. 'Scopolamine', (Roche).
The actions of this drug are similar to that of atropine, other than that the blocking effect on the vagus is said to be less. Although it has been used for premedication in cats and dogs (doses 0.01 to 0.02 mg/kg), its variable effects on the central nervous system limit its use.

SEDATION

Simple definitions.

A Tranquilliser: relieves anxiety, tension and inhibitions, without causing drowsiness.

A Sedative: also calms the patients but causes drowsiness.

A Hypnotic: will induce sleep from which it is possible to arouse the patient.

Further depression of the central nervous system leads to basal narcosis and to general anaesthesia.

These definitions are over simplified and most drugs fall into more than one category, depending on the dose rates used. Recent terminology has re-defined the drugs as anti-anxiety, antipsychotic, or sedative/hypnotic, but even with these new definitions, drugs fall into more than one category. However, a knowledge of which class of drug fits most closely, will often explain the limitations and reasons for failure in its use.

General comments.

In all animals, sedative type drugs are most effective if the patient is left quietly whilst induction occurs. Even following I/V administration, a short period of calm is required. In man, tranquillisation without drowsiness is usually required, but the veterinary surgeon often needs control, so that sedation is more important. However, if the drug used has tranquillising properties and relieves anxiety, it is effective in obtaining sedation in the nervous patient, but ineffective in the vicious animal. Also, if the patient is in pain, then sedation will not occur unless analgesics are also administered.

DRUGS USED TO SEDATE ANIMALS

PHENOTHIAZINES

These drugs are primarily tranquillising agents and indeed, in man, are now mainly used to treat psychosis, sedation being considered an unwanted side effect. Increasing the dose of phenothiazine drugs does not increase sedation and eventually results in Parkinson-type tremors. In animals, when used at the optimal dose, drugs of this class can provide effective sedation in nervous patients, but where sedation does not occur, then other sedatives or drug combinations must be employed.

Acepromazine 'ACP', (C-Vet), 'BK-Ace', (BK Veterinary Products)

For small animal use, this is available as a 2 mg/ml solution for injection and in tablet forms for oral use.

The general properties significant during clinical use include:-

a. tranquillisation and sedation
b. anti-emetic
c. spasmolytic
d. antihistamine (very weak action)
e. hypotension and adrenergic block

Side effects.

These are mainly due to the adrenergic block, which result in hypotension, excessive vagal tone and bradycardia. The bradycardia may be controlled with atropine. Some breeds, particularly Boxers, are excessively sensitive and may faint following the use of even fairly low doses. Hypovolaemic patients also respond by a severe fall in blood pressure and cardiovascular collapse. Where dehydration is suspected, it is advisable to insert an indwelling intravenous catheter before acepromazine is administered, as it may be difficult to catheterise the vein once hypotension is present. Treatment of hypotension consists of fluid replacement and the use, if necessary, of vasopressor drugs such as noradrenaline.

Acepromazine lowers the threshold in epileptic cases and may predispose to convulsions. In the author's experience this effect is restricted to higher doses than those recommended below.

Use as a Tranquilliser and Sedative.

In most animals, acepromazine causes tranquillisation with moderate sedation. The dose/response relationship for sedation levels out rapidly so that, after a certain point, higher dosage increases side effects without affecting sedation. There is, therefore, no point in using higher doses of acepromazine. There are individual animals in which it is impossible to obtain sedation with phenothiazine drugs and for those, a narcotic analgesic should be added (i.e. giving a neuroleptanalgesic mixture), or another class of sedative should be used. On average, nervous or sick animals respond well to acepromazine, whilst vicious animals do not. It is also less effective as a sedative in cats than in dogs.

Use as Premedication.

The sedative and anti-emetic properties of acepromazine make it a useful premedicant drug in dogs and to a lesser extent in cats. Acepromazine premedication increases the length of action of subsequent anaesthetic drugs and also reduces the barbiturate required for induction by about one third.

Other uses.

These include oral use as an anti-emetic against sickness and at very low doses, for tranquillisation without sedation in behavioural problems.

Routes of administration and dose rates.

Dogs.

a. I/M injection: **0.03–0.2 mg/kg.**
b. I/V injection: at lower end of I/M range.
   N.B. After I/V administration it may take 10 minutes or more for the drug to exert its full effect.
   The I/V route should be avoided in hypotensive or hypovolaemic patients.
c. Oral route: 1–3 mg/kg.
d. Subcutaneous route: widely used, although less reliable than I/M.

Please note: The lowest levels quoted for intramuscular and intravenous use are considerably lower than those which have been quoted by the manufacturer. They are, however, adequate for premedication in most dogs and, particularly in the larger breeds, which seem to be very sensitive to acepromazine, and will often produce maximal sedation.

Cats.

In cats, sedation is much less reliable and is rarely adequate for anything other than premedication. For this purpose doses of 0.1 to 0.2 mg/kg by I/M injection are usually used.

Other Phenothiazines used in veterinary practice include:

Chlorpromazine 'Largactil'

Methotrimeprazine 'in Small Animal Immobilon'

Proprionyl promazine 'Combelene', widely used in other European countries

Promazine 'Sparine'

Promethazine 'Phenergan' — used as an antihistamine rather than a sedative

Trimeprazine 'Vallergan'

BUTYROPHENONES

Droperidol 'Droleptan', (Janssen Pharmaceutica)

Fluanisone

Azaperone 'Suicalm', 'Stresnil', (Janssen Pharmaceutica)

Droperidol and fluanisone are used in dogs in the neuroleptanalgesic mixtures, 'Innovar-Vet' and 'Hypnorm', because of their potent action in preventing opiate-induced vomiting. They do not depress respiration, but do cause moderate hypotension. Little has been reported on the clinical use of butyrophenones alone in dogs, but following the use of the neuroleptanalgesic mixture 'Innovar' in dogs, there have been reports of aggressive behaviour for up to 48 hours following sedation. In man, although the drugs cause apparent tranquillisation and cataleptic immobility, this may mask severe mental restlessness and distress. Intravenous use of azaperone in both pigs and horses causes violent excitement in a high proportion of cases and restlessness is a feature of the induction phase following intramuscular use of this drug in pigs. If these properties also occur in small animals, it would seem that other agents will be preferable for sedation in these species.

ALPHA 2 ADRENOCEPTOR AGONISTS DRUGS AND THEIR ANTAGONISTS

Xylazine has been used as a sedative in veterinary medicine since 1968, but its mode of action was not originally understood. It is now known that it acts by specifically stimulating alpha 2 adrenoceptors. Recently medetomidine, a more potent alpha 2 adrenoceptor agonist, has become available as a sedative for cats and dogs. Both these drugs are potent sedatives and analgesics, but also have many side effects.

The effects of alpha 2 adrenoceptor agonists can be reversed by the use of specific alpha 2 adrenoceptor antagonists, such as atipamezole and yohimbine.

ALPHA 2 ADRENOCEPTOR AGONISTS

Use as sedatives/hypnotics.

Xylazine and medetomidine both produce marked sedation and analgesia which are dose dependent up to a maximum effect after which increasing dose increases the duration of action. At high doses depth of sedation may be adequate to allow a wide range of procedures, but the animals are **not** anaesthetised; are capable of arousal, and should therefore be handled with normal precautions. Additional analgesia (e.g. local analgesia or general anaesthesia) is required for surgical procedures. If the mouth is to be examined a secure, effective gag should be utilised. Sedation is most satisfactory if the animal is calm before drug administration, and adequate time must be allowed for the drug to have full effect before manipulations are commenced. Combinations with opioid drugs increase the degree of sedation achieved.

Use as Premedication.

Medetomidine and xylazine are useful premedicant agents, and are particularly effective in reducing the muscular hypertonicity caused by ketamine anaesthesia. However, they markedly reduce the dose required of any subsequent anaesthetic (intravenous or inhalation) and **special care** is required to avoid anaesthetic overdose. The extent of this reduction is generally dependent on the dose of the sedative agent, but even in apparently poorly sedated animals there are marked anaesthetic-sparing effects. Following xylazine or medetomidine sedation, there is a considerable delay (sometimes over one minute) between the intravenous injection of an anaesthetic agent and its effects becoming apparent. If this fact is not appreciated it is easy to overdose. The uptake of inhalation agents is also delayed.

Following sedation with xylazine or medetomidine superficial veins are often difficult to visualise. Where practical, the prior placement of a venous catheter allows easy administration of subsequent intravenous drugs.

Side effects.

In small animals, both xylazine and medetomidine cause bradycardia and a fall in cardiac output. Blood pressure is slightly reduced, although there may be an early hypertensive phase. Atropine will reverse the bradycardia, but this is not always beneficial, the combination of atropine often results in severe cardiac arrythmias and/or marked hypertension. Xylazine has been shown to reduce the threshold for the production of adrenaline induced cardiac arrhythmias. In deeply sedated dogs and cats respiration may become intermittent in nature, and some animals show slight cyanosis. Hypothermia may result from prolonged sedation. Other side effects include vomiting on induction (less common after medetomidine), slight muscular tremors, reduced intestinal motility and increased uterine contraction. Hormonal effects include inhibition of insulin release (resulting in hyperglycaemia) and a decrease in ADH (causing marked diuresis).

Contraindications and special warnings.

Alpha 2 adrenoceptor agonists should only be used with great caution in animals with cardiopulmonary disease or which are suffering from dehydration. Xylazine is specifically contraindicated in the last stages of pregnancy and, although medetomidine has a lesser effect on the uterus, the manufacturers currently do not advise its use in pregnant animals. The effects on insulin release and blood glucose levels must be considered in animals suffering from diabetes mellitus. If sedation is being used to aid clinical investigation, care must be taken to ensure the side effects are considered in interpretation of results.

Xylazine. 'Rompun' (Bayer). 'Anased' (BK Products).

Dose rates recommended for dogs and cats are from 1-3 mg/kg I/M or S/C, although subcutaneous administration is less reliable. Emesis may occur during induction of sedation, and is most common following the lower doses. Maximal sedation is achieved within 20 minutes of I/M injection and after 3mg/kg, lasts for about 1 hour, sedation gradually lightening over the next hour. When used as a premedicant, xylazine reduces the doses of thiopentone or 'Saffan' subsequently required by at least a half.

Medetomidine. 'Domitor' (SmithKline, Beecham).

In dogs, the licensed doses of medetomidine are 10-80 µg/kg by I/V, I/M or S/C injection, the lower doses being advised for premedication. Even lower doses (5µg/kg) produce a calming effect. Sedation is dose-dependent up to a maximum (usually achieved within 15 minutes of 40 µg/kg I/M or within 5 minutes of 20 µg/kg I/V), duration at this dose being from 1-2 hours. Higher doses give prolonged effects. Subcutaneous administration is less reliable. Dosage is best calculated on a surface-area rather than a weight basis; practically, this meaning that small dogs (less than 10 kg bwt.) require higher doses than large dogs. Emesis does occur during induction but less commonly than after xylazine, and is rare following I/V injection. Medetomidine is absorbed across mucous membranes and has been used effectively by 'squirting' into the mouth. It is inactivated in the stomach, so is ineffective given on food.

Cats are more resistant to the effects of medetomidine, and licensed doses in this species are 50-150 µg/kg by I/M or S/C injection. Doses of 80 µg/kg I/M produce deep sedation, which may be very prolonged. Care must be taken to avoid hypothermia. Vomiting during induction occurs more commonly than in dogs.

In both cats and dogs, when medetomidine is used for premedication, it results in a dose-related reduction of subsequent anaesthetic required. In deeply sedated animals minimal anaesthetic agent may be required. For example, in dogs given 40 µg/kg medetomidine I/M doses of 1 mg/kg propofol or 2 mg/kg thiopentone are adequate for anaesthetic induction, and in cats give 80-100 µg/kg medetomidine I/M, ketamine at doses of 2.5-5 mg/kg I/M results in good anaesthesia with excellent relaxation.

The data sheet recommends the use of gloves when handling medetomidine.

Detomidine. 'Domosedan' (SmithKline, Beecham).

This drug is currently licensed in the UK for use in horses only. Detomidine is **not** recommended for use in small animals.

ALPHA 2 ADRENOCEPTOR ANTAGONISTS.

These antagonists reverse the sedative and the majority of the side effects of xylazine and of medetomidine. Although several such drugs exist (e.g. yohimbine, idazoxan), currently the only one available for veterinary use in the UK is atipamezole.

Atipamezole. 'Antisedan' (SmithKline, Beecham).

Atipamezole is a very potent specific alpha 2 antagonist which is licensed for use as an antagonist to medetomidine. For use in the dog the manufacturers have arranged that the concentration of 'Antisedan' (5 mg/ml atipamezole) is such that equal volumes to the original 'Domitor' (1 mg/ml medetomidine) used are required for reversal. Following the I/M injection of atipamezole to the medetomidine-sedated dog, arousal occurs within 3-7 minutes, and by 10 minutes the dog appears clinically normal. Arousal can be sudden, and it is advisable to have the dog positioned where it cannot fall (i.e. not on the table). At these doses cardiopulmonary depression is only partly antagonised, and pulse rates, though improved, remain lower than normal.

For the cat, lower doses (half the volume of Antisedan to the original Domitor) are recommended, as at the higher doses some cats appear hyperalert. Except in emergency atipamezole should not be given to the cat by the I/V route.

Although not licensed for the purpose, atipamazole at doses of 200 μg/kg has been used in the dog to reverse xylazine (3 mg/kg) sedation. Similarly, atipamezole has been used by the I/V route when rapid reversal has been required.

Atipamezole has no effect on any residual anaesthetic drugs. Thus, if used when medetomidine has been used for premedication, arousal will depend on the remaining anaesthetic agents present. Where medetomidine/ketamine combinations have been employed, atipamezole should not be given until the effects of the ketamine have waned.

The Data sheet recommends the use of gloves when handling atipamezole.

Other properties, however, are similar and reports of its use are as follows:-

> **Premedication.** Sedation is minimal and the removal of anxieties and inhibitions often make the domestic pet more difficult to control. The quantity of anaesthetic required following its use is very little reduced, but sleeping times are considerably lengthened. It is useful for its anticonvulsant and muscle relaxant properties e.g.:-
>
> a. prior to ketamine anaesthesia
> b. prior to myelography. Suggested dose for dog : 5—20 mg I/M.
>
> **Post operative restlessness.** Provided pain is relieved by analgesics, diazepam at up to 1 mg/kg slowly, as required I/V, is very effective at relieving post operative restlessness. The maximum suggested dose is up to 5 mg/kg hour.
>
> **Anticonvulsant and Anti-epileptic.**
> **Dogs:** up to 5 mg slowly I/V, repeated, if necessary, after 2 minutes, is reported to stop the convulsions in a high percentage of cases.
> **Cats:** use of from 2 mg to 10 mg slowly I/V or I/M, has been reported for severe convulsions.
>
> **Psychotic effects.** Small doses orally, have been used to control behavioural problems in dogs.
>
> **Appetite stimulant.** Very low doses have been used for this purpose, especially in cats.

Other benzodiazepines in veterinary use include **midazolam** 'Hypnovel', (Roche), a water soluble form of benzodiazepine that is suitable for I/V use. In small animals, it has been used primarily as part of anaesthetic combinations. **Zolazepam** is used in combination with the dissociative anaesthetic agent, tiletamine.

BENZODIAZEPINE ANTAGONISTS

> **Flumazenil** 'Anexzate', (Roche).
> This benzodiazepine antagonist has recently been licenced for use in man. In the dog, it has been used (in combination with naloxone), to reverse anaesthesia induced with benzodiazepine/opioid combinations.

SEDATIVE/OPIOID COMBINATIONS

When sedative and opioid drugs are combined, their actions are synergistic, sedation and analgesia being more intense than the sum of that produced by either drug alone. Such combinations have been used for many years, but became fashionable in the 1950's with the development of neuroleptanalgesia.

Neuroleptanalgesia

This involves the combination of a potent opioid analgesic with a neuroleptic (anti psychotic agent). The phenothiazine and butyrophenone drugs are neuroleptic agents. The degree of sedation and analgesia achieved depends on the drugs and the dosage used. It can vary from deep sedation to a state equal to full anaesthesia where there is unconsciousness with intense analgesia. This latter state is termed neuroleptanaesthesia.

In man, the preferred technique consists of the prior administration of the neuroleptic agent, followed by the analgesic given I/V to effect. The use of potent analgesics in this way, cause respiratory depression and ventilation is assisted, if necessary. This technique can be applied in the dog and gives very satisfactory results. In general, veterinary surgeons prefer to administer mixtures of the two drugs together. However, this gives less controllable results, and the chance of overdose when the potent opioids are used, is higher.

Opioids may also be used in combination with benzodiazepine or with alpha 2 adrenoceptor agonist sedative drugs. These combinations can not technically be called neuroleptanalgesic mixtures, but the principle of use is similar.

General precautions.

Combinations incorporating the more potent opioids (e.g. fentanyl, etorphine), are not used in cats as they may induce excitement. Similarly, no opioid combination should be used I/V in this species. The depth of sedation produced by some of these combinations can be intense, and may be associated with respiratory depression. The degree of monitoring and of care required by the patient is similar to that required after the administration of a general anaesthetic.

'Homemade' combinations.

Many sedative/opioid combinations have been utilised, but few have been well assessed for efficacy or for pharmacological effects. The following combinations includes those with which authors of this book have experience, but the list is not comprehensive. N.B. Of the opioids mentioned in the 'homemade combinations' below, only pethidine and butorphanol are licenced for veterinary use in the U.K.

Phenothiazine combinations.

    A. Acepromazine/omnopon/scopolamine. I/M.

        The dose for a large dog (35 kg or above) would be 20 mg omnopon, 0.4 mg scopolamine and 2–3 mg acepromazine, given together by I/M injection. This will give reasonable sedation to allow easy handling in the most vicious dog. Vomiting often occurs. Analgesia is not sufficient to allow surgery.

    B. Acepromazine/pethidine. I/M.

        Acepromazine at 0.07 mg/kg and pethidine at 3 mg/kg I/M gives good sedation for radiographic procedures.
        I/V route. Lower doses are required. Acepromazine at 0.05 mg/kg and pethidine at 1-2 mg/kg are effective. However, intravenous pethidine can cause severe hypotension.

    C. Acepromazine/buprenorphine. I/M.

        Acepromazine at 0.05-0.7 mg/kg and buprenorphine at 9-10 μg/kg I/M, give effective sedation for radiography.

    D. Propionyl promazine/methadone.

        This mixture is widely used for sedation and premedication in other European countries and is indeed, available there as a commercial combination 'Combelene Polamivet'.

Alpha 2 adrenoceptor agonist combinations.

    A. Xylazine/methadone.

        In Europe, other than the UK, these drugs are often used in combination.

B. Medetomidine/butorphanol. I/M.

Sedation produced by medetomidine 40 µg/kg I/M plus butorphanol, 0.05 mg/kg I/M, is considerably deeper than that produced by the same dose of medetomidine alone.

COMMERCIAL MIXTURES

The following commercial neuroleptanalgesic mixtures are available.

1. Hypnorm (Janssen Pharmaceutica)

Contains: Fentanyl 0.315 mg/ml
Fluanisone 10 mg/ml

When given either intravenously or subcutaneously to dogs, it produces a deep sedation and excellent analgesia very rapidly, the effects being at their peak within 15 minutes. It is used for premedication prior to full general anaesthetic (when the dose of other anaesthetics given should be minimal), or on its own for sedation and anaesthesia for minor surgery. Side effects include bradycardia (counteracted by atropine), defaecation, hypersensitivity to sound, and variable respiratory depression. These respiratory effects make it contra-indicated in respiratory disease and it is also contra-indicated in cases of advanced renal and liver failure. Its action may, if necessary, be reversed by naloxone, but the short action of fentanyl (30 minutes), usually makes it unnecessary, although the action of fluanisone persists for some time.

Hypnorm has also been used very successfully in a variety of small mammals including guinea pigs and rabbits (see chapter 17).

2. Immobilon S.A. (C-Vet Ltd)

Contains: Etorphine hydrochloride 0.074 mg/ml
Methotrimeprazine 18 mg/ml

This can be administered by the intramuscular or intravenous routes to obtain very deep sedation, hypnosis and intense analgesia, which is adequate for many minor to moderate surgical procedures. Surgical analgesia lasts from 1 to 1 ½ hours and further doses can be given. Side effects may include severe respiratory depression resulting in cyanosis, bradycardia and hypotension. In particular, in older dogs, the aged metabolic systems may be further damaged by hypoxia, so such patients should be given oxygen supplementation, assisted ventilation and treatment for hypotension should these side effects occur.

The use of diprenorphine 'Revivon SA' reverses the action of etorphine and rouses the dog, although moderate sedation remains from the effect of the neuroleptic. The manfacturers have arranged that the concentration of 'Revivon SA' is such that an equal volume of Revivon to that of 'Immobilon' originally is given is required. Some dogs relapse into sleep again 4-8 hours later, but will re-awake with a further dose of diprenorphine.

When 'Immobilon' is followed by the use of general anaesthetic, very small doses of anaesthetic are required. Severe respiratory depression may occur and if troublesome, may be reversed by diprenorphine.

Immobilon. Emergency procedure in man.

Man is very susceptible to 'Immobilon', not only by injection, but also by absorption through cuts or mucous membranes and those using it should ensure that they, and their lay staff, are familiar with the procedure for handling the drug and for emergency treatment in man, as printed on each box of the drug.

Naloxone, or other narcotic antagonists suitable for use in man, should always be immediately available (i.e. out of the cupboard and at hand) whenever 'Immobilon' is used.

N.B. As 'Immobilon' is so potent, great care must be taken over the disposal of used syringes and needles.

SEDATION FOR RADIOGRAPHY

Restraint for radiography, radiotherapy or similar procedures require that the animal can be positioned, traction applied where necessary, and that the animal will remain immobile for several minutes (and in some cases, longer). This can be achieved by general anaesthesia. However, sedatives or sedative combinations are often used in order to avoid giving an anaesthetic. In some cases, this is very satisfactory, but where deep sedation is necessary, the animal may be compromised to a greater degree than it would be by a well administered anaesthetic. Full facilities for resuscitation are still necessary and the sedated patients require careful monitoring until full recovery.

In general, acepromazine and the alpha 2 agonist sedative drugs given alone, or in the combinations already discussed, prove satisfactory for sedation for radiography. However, the following points should be considered when deciding on the method to be used.

> In all cases ensuring that the animal is comfortable (using suitable pads etc) reduces the sedation that is required. Often, when first positioned, the animal tries to move, but if gently restrained for a short time, will settle and tolerate the procedure with no further sedation being required. Quiet surroundings are essential for any sedative to be effective.

> It is important that the animal does not become hypersensitive to sound. The commercial neuroleptic mixtures such as Hypnorm, tend to have this effect.

> The drugs utilised for sedation must not effect the result of the investigations to be carried out (e.g. the alpha 2 agonists and some of the opioids affect gut motility).

> Acepromazine may give sufficient sedation on its own but if positioning is difficult, acepromazine/opiate combinations such as acepromazine/pethidine, or acepromazine/buprenorphine, have proved very satisfactory. These combinations do cause some respiratory depression.

> In fit animals, xylazine or medetomidine usually give adequate sedation for radiography. If inadequate, combinations with opioids may be used. Occasionally, muscles twitches can prove awkward. The length of action is prolonged compared with the procedure required, but antagonists to these sedatives such as atipamezole are now available for clinical use. These drugs are best avoided in sick animals because of the cardiovascular side effects.

FURTHER READING

HALL, L. W. and CLARKE, K. W. (1991). *Veterinary Anaesthesia,* 9th ed. Balliere Tindall.

CLARKE, K. W. and ENGLAND, G. C. W. (1989). *Medetomidine, a new sedative analgesic for use in the dog and its reversal by atipamezole.* J. Small An. Prac. **30,** 343-348.

LEES, P. (1991). Chapter 20 in *Veterinary Applied Pharmacology and Therapeutics.* Ed. Brander, G. C., Pugh, D. M., Bywater, R. J. and Jenkins, W. L. Balliere Tindall, London.

LIVINGSTON, A., NOLAN, A. and WATERMAN, A. E. (1986/87). *The pharmacology of adrenergic agonist drugs.* J. Assoc. Vet. Anaesth. **14,** 3-10.

TAYLOR, P. M. and HERRTAGE, M. E. (1986). *Evaluation of some drug combinations.* J. Small An. Prac. **27,** 325-333.

CHAPTER 6

INTRAVENOUS ANAESTHESIA

A. E. Waterman B.V.Sc., Ph.D., D.V.A., M.R.C.V.S.
J. N. Lucke B.V.Sc., Ph.D., D.V.A., M.R.C.V.S.

INTRODUCTION

INDICATIONS

1. For induction of anaesthesia to be followed by inhalational agents.
2. As a sole anaesthetic agent for short term minor procedures such as radiography, suturing, suture removal or ear examination.
3. As a supplement to inhalation anaesthesia.
4. To aid in the treatment of conditions such as tetanus and status epilepticus.

Advantages	Disadvantages
Simple	Superficial vein may be difficult to find
Rapid onset of anaesthesia	Animal may struggle
Relatively pleasant for animal	Drug may be irritant if given perivascularly
No apparatus needed	Once injected it cannot be removed
No explosion/pollution hazard	Drug may be cumulative
Non-irritant to airways	If the animal is not intubated, you are not ready for a respiratory emergency
	Possible excitement in recovery
	Possible apnoea on injection

Techniques

As a single dose
By topping up with increments
As a continuous infusion

PRACTICAL ASPECTS OF INTRAVENOUS INJECTION

Proper pre-anaesthetic medication should preclude the necessity for forceful restraint for intravenous injection. In seriously debilitated or aged animals when premedication is deemed unwise, gentle handling by a competent assistant should be all that is required.

It is helpful to position the animal on a non-slip surface either on a table or the floor depending on the size of the patient.

Site.

The easiest vein for injection is the cephalic (radial vein). The recurrent tarsal (saphenous) vein may be used, but restraint is more difficult and the animal's response to the anaesthetic agent cannot be observed so easily. The external jugular vein is not recommended for injection unless it is catheterised, since it is much more difficult to ensure that all the drug is deposited slowly intravenously, therefore, there is a tendency to administer drugs too rapidly by this route.

Equipment.

For a single injection, a suitable gauge hypodermic needle will suffice but if repeated injections or an infusion are contemplated, an over the needle catheter should be used. This will ensure that the vein is not damaged and the drug is not injected perivascularly. There is a wide variety of teflon catheters available and choice depends on personal preference. However, it is worth emphasising that for successful placement of these, it is best to make a small nick in the skin so that the point of the catheter is not damaged as it passes through the skin. As the inner needle enters the vein, blood 'flashes back' into the hub of the catheter, which should then be advanced into the vein while the needle is held firmly.
The catheter must then be secured firmly by adhesive tape.

CLASSES OF DRUGS

1. BARBITURATES
2. STEROIDS
3. DISSOCIATIVE AGENTS
4. PROPOFOL
5. NEUROLEPTANAESTHETICS

1. BARBITURATES

These are given I/V only.

Drugs:
Thiopentone Sodium
Methohexitone Sodium
Pentobarbitone Sodium

a. **THIOPENTONE SODIUM,** 'Intraval', (May & Baker).

Thiopentone sodium is still the 'bench mark' for other I/V agents. It is a short acting thiobarbiturate supplied as a powder. Once made up with sterile water, the solution is stable for 3—7 days depending on temperature. The solution is very alkaline (pH 14) and, therefore, irritant if the concentration is greater than 2.5%. The solution is not miscible with acidic drugs as precipitation occurs.

Actions

i. Rapid onset of unconsciousness but at sub-anaesthetic concentrations all barbiturates are hyperalgesic (i.e. reduce the pain threshold).

ii. Thiopentone produces dose related respiratory depression and apnoea occasionally occurs at induction, especially if the drug is administered rapidly. If apnoea occurs, oxygen should be administered and I.P.P.V. instituted.

iii. The cardiovascular system is depressed so that after injection there is hypotension and secondary tachycardia. Myocardial contractility is depressed and coronary perfusion is impaired temporarily. These cardiovascular effects are of significance only in hypovolaemic animals or those with heart disease.

Pharmacology

Thiopentone sodium is a highly lipid soluble, weak organic acid and is a highly protein bound (approx 75% in dogs) drug. As with all anaesthetic drugs, only the unbound, un-ionised fraction of the drug is able to penetrate cell membranes and thus produce its effect. Therefore, the response to a given dose of the drug will vary depending on the pH of the blood (normally 39% is ionised but this percentage decreases as pH falls and an acidosis will enhance penetration of the blood brain barrier) and on the concentration of plasma proteins. Hypoproteinaemia or uraemia (which results in displacement of the drug from binding sites) will also increase the percentage of unbound and, therefore, active drug.

The high lipid solubility of thiopentone favours the rapid onset of unconsciousness within one circulation time (20–30 seconds). Delay in onset of unconsciousness will occur if the circulation is slowed by disease or age.

Following a single injection of thiopentone, plasma levels decline rapidly in either a biexponential or triexponential manner, as the drug is redistributed from the brain to other tissues of the body (the distribution half-life is around 6 to 15 minutes in dogs). Initially, the drug is taken up by relatively well perfused tissue (muscles) and later by the lipid tissue which is less well perfused and in which the uptake is slower. Thiopentone is metabolised slowly by the liver, but the rate is so slow as to contribute only insignificantly to recovery from a single dose of the drug. However, ultimately all the administered drug is metabolised before excretion. (The half-life of the elimination phase is 7 hours.) It is clear then that the duration of effect approximates to distribution rather than elimination.

Clinical Relevance of Pharmacokinetics

i.   Small doses rapidly induce a brief period of anaesthesia.

ii. Incremental doses will result in saturation of the vessel rich and vessel poor tissues (muscle and fat), so that recovery will then depend solely on metabolism, which is slow.

iii. Dogs which are thin, emaciated, hypoproteinaemic (liver disease), or uraemic, all show an increased sensitivity to a single dose as more of the given dose is active.

iv. Certain breeds (greyhound family), show a markedly delayed recovery from the effects of thiopentone. This is generally attributed to their low body fat to lean mass ratio.

v.   Large doses of the drug will not only delay recovery but will also, by virtue of its ant-analgesic effect, produce restlessness and an increased requirement for analgesia for as long as 7 hours (the elimination half-life of the drug in dogs).

Use

The drug should be used as a 2.5% or 1% solution to minimise the risk of causing damage, should it seep peri-vascularly and also to enable accurate administration, especially to small dogs and cats.

It is important to give the drug 'to effect' and not to give a computed dose since each individual will vary as to its requirements. However, as a guide, in unpremedicated fit animals, a dose of around 20–25 mg/kg may be required to produce unconsciousness sufficient to permit endotracheal intubation. This dose is halved by the use of premedication agents. The dose should be given slowly (over 30–40 seconds) so that the injection may be stopped once the desired effect is obtained. An even slower rate of injection should be used in sick animals (60 seconds or more). In cats it may be necessary to give the drug slightly more quickly since they tend to struggle more while being restrained.

Problems

i.   Peri-vascular injection of the drug in large volumes or high concentrations (>2.5%) will cause a marked reaction with phlebitis, inflammation and even necrosis of surrounding tissues. Any suspected leakage should be treated immediately by the infiltration of large volumes of sterile saline (up to 20 ml) to which 1–2 ml of 2% lignocaine or 5% procaine may be added. Failure to institute such measures, not only subjects the animal to needless suffering, but may be construed as negligence.

b. **METHOHEXITONE SODIUM** 'Brietal' (Elanco Products)

An oxybarbiturate supplied as a powder. When made up in sterile water, it is relatively stable for about six weeks. It is used as a 1% solution, which is less irritant, if inadvertently injected perivascularly, than thiopentone.

Its actions are similar to thiopentone but there are differences:
i. It is less protein bound, less ionised at body pH (24%) and, therefore, more of a given dose is effective..
ii. It is slightly less lipid soluble, therefore, more drug stays in the central compartment and is available for extraction and metabolism by the liver.
iii. Its rate of intrinsic hepatic clearance is greater (i.e. it is metabolised at a faster rate).
iv. Its potency is approximately twice that of thiopentone.

The net result of the above is that recovery from anaesthesia is slightly faster with less hangover and a shorter period of ant-analgesia.

v. Apnoea after induction is more common.
vi. Muscle spasms are more common at both induction and recovery.

Use.

It should be given 'to effect' as for thiopentone. On average, approximately 5 mg/kg is required to produce unconsciousness in premedicated animals, but it is best to give approximately half this and then top up, incrementally, to effect.

The drug may also be given by infusion or incrementally without prolonging recovery. Approximately 0.3 mg/kg/min as a 0.1% solution will generally maintain anaesthesia.

Methohexitone does not cause prolonged recovery in greyhounds and related breeds and is, therefore, preferred to thiopentone for these animals.

c. **PENTOBARBITONE SODIUM** 'Sagatal' (RMB)

This is one of the oldest intravenous anaesthetic drugs. It is an oxybarbiturate similar in structure to thiopentone. It is available as a 6% solution which is relatively non-irritant.

Pharmacology
i. Pentobarbitone has a slow onset of action (at least 60–90 seconds) because it takes time to cross the blood-brain barrier. This is due to its low lipid solubility (1/16 thiopentone) and a lower permeability coefficient into CSF, (0.17 versus 0.5 for thiopentone).
ii. It is less protein bound (40%) and less ionised (17%) at normal blood pH than thiopentone, so a greater proportion stays in the central compartment.
iii. It has a long duration of action because metabolism, which is relatively slow, is its main route of clearance from the body. Its low lipid solubility precludes any significant degree of redistribution and, thus, recovery is related to its elimination half-life, which is 200 minutes in dogs.

Clinical Relevance
i. Both induction and recovery are prolonged, therefore, excitement and ant-analgesia are common since they occur during periods of light narcosis.
ii. Respiratory depression is marked and prolonged and attempts to use this drug as a sole anaesthetic agent are extremely hazardous since concentrations sufficient to produce a depth of anaesthesia suitable to perform surgery will often lead to hypoventilation that will be very marked once surgical stimulation ceases.
iii. Cardiovascular depression is also marked.
iv. Hypothermia is common in the prolonged recovery period following the use of this drug. This sets up a vicious circle in which hypothermia reduces the rate of hepatic metabolism of the drug, which further delays recovery, which therefore predisposes to hypothermia.

Use

The prolonged duration of recovery and marked ant-analgesic effect of this drug means that it cannot be recommended for use as a sole anaesthetic agent in any but the fittest dogs and even then, additional inspired oxygen (30%) should be provided and special measures instituted to prevent post-operative hypothermia. Its use in cats and very small dogs cannot, in any case, be recommended since recovery is very prolonged and morbidity will be higher in these animals.

Fit healthy dogs

An approximate dose of 25—30 mg/kg is calculated but, as with all drugs, the agent must be given to effect. The dose rate may be reduced considerably by the judicious use of premedication agents such as acepromazine. In small dogs it is safer to dilute the drug to a 3% solution and to use a fine gauge needle so that it cannot be injected too quickly. Half to two-thirds of the computed dose should be given over 15 seconds in order to avoid a period of excitement. It takes 1.5 to 2 minutes before the full effects of the dose are seen and the rest of the dose should therefore be injected slowly over a further 3—4 minutes until the animal is unconscious, but still has a sluggish pedal reflex. If anaesthesia is deepened beyond this level, the degree of respiratory and cardiovascular depression produced is too dangerous. If the procedure cannot then be carried out under pentobarbitone alone, it is better to use supplementary drugs such as local anaesthetic agents or inhalational agents, than to inject more pentobarbitone.

Cats

Although this drug has been used in the past, there are now far better agents available and its use cannot be advocated because of the extremely prolonged recovery and consequent severe hypothermia and hypoxia produced in cats.

2. STEROIDS

a. **ALPHAXALONE/ALPHADOLONE ACETATE** 'Saffan', (Pitman Moore)

'Saffan' is a mixture of two steroid agents; alphaxalone (9 mg/ml) and alphadolone acetate (3 mg/ml). These drugs are not water soluble and are, therefore, solubilised by the use of 20% 'Cremophor EL.' (polyoxyethylated castor oil). The solution is clear but viscous and of a neutral pH. Once opened, the vials (5 or 10 ml) should be used at once since there is no bacteriostatic agent included in the preparation. Do not store in the refrigerator as the steroids tend to precipitate out of solution. The solution is non-irritant if injected perivascularly.

Dogs

The drug is not licenced for use in dogs, which may exhibit a marked anaphylactic reaction to 'Cremophor EL'. This can be fatal, therefore, it is not safe to use the drug in dogs. The reported use of the drug, in combination with large doses of antihistamines, seems an unnecessary and dangerous choice when other, safer, drugs are available.

Cats

Pharmacology

i. These agents have no hormonal effects.

ii. Induction time is roughly the same as for thiopentone if the drug is given I/V.

iii. Both components are metabolised rapidly by the liver. The duration of action of a single dose of the drug is therefore very short and recovery is rapid; except that in cats with hepatic dysfunction, metabolism is likely to be delayed and the drug will have a prolonged duration of action. Renal dysfunction will also delay the excretion of metabolites slightly and may affect recovery.

iv. The drugs are only 30—50% protein bound, therefore, the effects of a given dose of 'Saffan', are likely to be less enhanced by the presence of hypoproteinaemia than would a comparable dose of a thiobarbiturate.

v. It has a wider safety margin than barbiturates in cats.

vi. It produces less apnoea at induction and less respiratory depression than barbiturates.

vii. It produces a dose related degree of cardiovascular depression with both hypotension and tachycardia being evident.

viii. Like all anaesthetic agents, 'Saffan' will cross the placenta and produce foetal depression. Its use should, therefore, be confined to the induction of anaesthesia only, in cats requiring caesarian section. Sufficient time should be allowed for redistribution of the drug from the kittens before they are delivered (see chapter 10).

ix. Anaphylactoid Reactions. Occasionally, 'Saffan' also causes histamine release in cats. The severity of these reactions varies from mild subcutaneous oedema of the paws and pinnae to more severe laryngeal and pulmonary oedema and profound hypotension. Although fatalities are rare, it is probably best to avoid using the drug when airway surgery is contemplated or if the animal has a history of atopy.

x. 'Saffan' is absorbed so slowly from subcutaneous sites of injection that adequate plasma levels are never achieved. Hence, the drug will be ineffective unless given either intramuscularly or intravenously.

Use in cats

Intramuscular

Inject into a suitable muscle mass. The quadriceps group is usually preferable to other leg muscles, which have more intermuscular spaces into which the drug may be deposited inadvertently and from which absorption will be so slow as to reduce the effectiveness of the drug.

Dose:

The intramuscular dose can range from 4 mg/kg (suitable for premedication before topping up by the I/V route some 10 minutes later), to 18 mg/kg which will induce full anaesthesia within 10—15 minutes. However, the highest dose represents a considerable volume (1.5 ml per kg) which can be difficult to inject. A median dose rate of around 9 mg/kg is used more usually, and this will produce sufficient control with the option of increasing the depth of anaesthesia by giving further drug intravenously.

Intravenous

As with all induction agents, 'Saffan' is best administered intravenously to effect.

Dose:

In healthy animals, approximately 6 mg/kg will induce anaesthesia sufficient to permit endotracheal intubation. For a short period of anaesthesia, sufficient for minor procedures (10 minutes), a further 3 mg/kg may be administered slowly until the desired depth of anaesthesia is achieved. In debilitated, or old animals, this further dose is not usually required.

Intermittent doses

If 'Saffan' is used as the sole anaesthetic agent, 0.5 ml increments may be injected as necessary to maintain anaesthesia or an infusion may be set up to deliver the drug at the rate of around 0.24 mg/kg/min.

Because the drug is eliminated rapidly by hepatic metabolism, repeated doses do not prolong recovery, which occurs within two hours or so, even following 24 hours anaesthesia/sedation, provided normal homeostasis has been maintained (i.e. fluid balance, acid base balance, respiratory function, cardiovascular stability and body temperature).

Problems

The use of barbiturates together, with 'Saffan', should be avoided as these drugs are likely to produce profound respiratory and cardiovascular depression if used together. It also makes sense to avoid the concurrent administration of other drugs which may have a cumulative depressant effect.

3. DISSOCIATIVE AGENTS

Dissociative agents produce a state of anaesthesia quite unlike that produced by the conventional drugs included in the rest of this chapter. All the drugs which may be classified as dissociative agents are phenylcyclohexylamines of which phencyclidine is the parent compound. Phenycyclidine is no longer manufactured except in South Africa from where it may be imported only for use by BVZS members in zoo animal work. There are two other members of this group of compounds which are worthy of mention, ketamine and tiletamine, both of which were developed by Parke-Davis.

a. **KETAMINE HCl** 'Vetalar', (Parke-Davis Veterinary Limited).

Ketamine HCl is presented in aqueous solution. It is a weak organic base and the HCl solution has a pH of 3.3—5.5 so that it is immiscible with alkaline solutions. The drug is formulated at a strength of 100 mg/ml in 5, 10 or 20 ml multi-dose vials. It is relatively stable for 3 years but bottles should be protected from light and excessive heat.

Pharmacology

i. Onset of anaesthesia is slow (1—2 minutes) even after I/V administration.

ii. Dissociative anaesthesia is a state whereby profound somatic analgesia is combined with a light plane of unconsciousness but the animal appears to be dissociated from its environment.

iii. The eyes remain open and laryngeal and swallowing reflexes tend to persist.

iv. Stimulation of the extra-pyramidal system occurs so that muscle tone is maintained or even enhanced.

v. Stimulation of the sympathetic system frequently leads to lacrimation and salivation.

vi. Cardiovascular effects are dose related. Central stimulation of the sympathetic system leads to a tachycardia and increase in blood pressure and cardiac output. Large doses given intravenously may produce a transient fall in blood pressure as the drug produces a direct but transient depression of the myocardium. Normally the hypertensive effects predominate unless very large doses are used. Peripheral resistance does not increase.

vii. The respiratory effects of ketamine in the dog and cat are interesting. There is a degree of respiratory depression initially and there is often periodic breath holding on inspiration giving rise to a so called 'apneustic' pattern of respiration. Generally, blood oxygen levels are well maintained (compared to barbiturates) and the good preservation of cardiac output allows tissue oxygenation to be well maintained.

viii. Ketamine is metabolised by the liver and both parent compound and metabolites are excreted in bile and via the kidneys. Hepatic dysfunction and renal disease will affect elimination of the drug and prolong its action considerably.

ix. Ketamine can produce tonic/clonic seizures in some felidae (particularly leopards) and canidae (4% incidence).

Clinical Use

Ketamine is licensed for use in both dogs and cats as well as in primates and the larger species (horses, calves).

The advantages of this drug include its potency, which means that only a small volume is required and the fact that it is effective whether given I/V, I/M or subcutaneously or even through the buccal mucosa.

The disadvantages centre on the very poor muscle relaxation achieved when the drug is used alone which makes its usefulness for surgery very limited. Because of this, the drug is nearly always used in combination with a sedative which is given to enhance muscle relaxation.

Cats

Alone

Ketamine can be used alone merely to provide restraint for handling (11–22 mg/kg I/M) while a larger dose (20–25 mg/kg I/M) will produce satisfactory restraint for minor surgery. If given intravenously, slightly less will be required (10–15 mg/kg).

Combinations

i. More commonly ketamine (20–25 mg/kg I/M) is combined with xylazine (1 mg/kg I/M) to provide a period of anaesthesia lasting some 30 minutes. The xylazine must be given about 20 minutes beforehand if the cat is not starved. The drugs may be given simultaneously in starved animals. Atropine should always be administered first (0.04 mg/kg) to counteract the cardiovascular effects of the xylazine and the salivation provoked by ketamine. Medetomidine may be used instead of xylazine in this combination, dose rates; Ketamine 5-7 mg/kg, medetomidine 80 µg/kg.

ii. Ketamine (20–25 mg/kg) may also be given together with acepromazine maleate (0.1 mg/kg I/M) and this combination again produces a reasonable quality of anaesthesia.

    After I/M administration, unconsciousness occurs within about 5 minutes and lasts around 30–40 minutes. Full recovery takes several hours (5–8 hours), especially if xylazine or medetomidine has been used, and hypothermia can be a problem. The use of atipamezole can therefore be advantageous in these cases.

Dogs

The high incidence of seizures encountered when ketamine is used alone in the dog, precludes its sole use.

Ketamine is only licensed for use in dogs (in the UK) in combination with xylazine.

Dose

Ketamine: 10 mg/kg I/M given 10 minutes after

Xylazine: 1–2 mg/kg I/M (lower dose in larger dogs).

It is probably advisable to reduce the dose rate of xylazine in older animals. Onset of anaesthesia occurs in 5–10 minutes and this combination provides approximately 30 minutes anaesthesia. Atropine should be given with the xylazine.

Alternatively, ketamine may be given intravenously at a dose rate of about 5 mg/kg following the administration of diazepam (0.1–0.2 mg/kg I/V). This combination provides quite smooth, slow induction of anaesthesia in debilitated animals. Salivation may occur but is rarely a major problem.

Problems

i.   Recovery from ketamine alone can be stormy, especially in cats. Disturbances such as noise, lights and handling may precipitate seizures.

ii. Hypothermia and delayed recovery may occur, especially in cats. It is important to keep the ambient temperature high in the recovery area.

iii. The depth of anaesthesia may be difficult to judge and inexperienced observers may conclude, wrongly, that supplementary drugs (including volatile agents) are required. Any additional anaesthetic drug will produce marked respiratory depression and must be administered with great care.

iv. Corneal drying may occur, the eyes should be protected by a bland ophthalmic ointment.

v.   The administration of xylazine or medetomidine in combination with ketamine carries the risk of vomiting at induction and this combination must not be used in cases with gastro-intestinal obstruction.

vi. The increase in blood pressure produced by ketamine makes it unsuitable for intraocular surgery (see chapter 12).

TILETAMINE

Tiletamine is chemically very closely related to ketamine in structure but is longer lasting, two or three times more potent and has more pronounced side effects (muscle rigidity and tonic/clonic seizures). It is, therefore, formulated in a preparation together with a benzodiazepine, zolazepam, which potentiates its anaesthetic effects while protecting against seizures and providing muscle relaxation.

The combination of tiletamine and zolezepan is being marketed as 'Zoletil' in Australia and 'Telazol' in the USA. It is not currently available in the UK but the situation may well change in the future.

Pharmacology

Its effects are similar to ketamine.

Dose of Combination

Dogs

I/M 7—15 mg/kg
I/V 5—10 mg/kg. } depending on the degree of restraint required.

Cats

I/M 10—15 mg/kg, onset 3—5 minutes.
I/V 5—7 mg/kg, onset 1 minute.

Always premedicate with atropine first.

The duration of anaesthesia is 20—60 minutes depending on the dose.

Full recovery takes up to 6 hours.

4. PROPOFOL

'Rapinovet', (Coopers Animal Health Limited), 'Diprivan' (I.C.I. Ltd.), is the medical product.

2,6 di-iso propyl phenol or I.C.I. 35868, is a simple chemical belonging to the class of compounds known as 'hindered phenols'.

This drug was developed by ICI Ltd. in 1980. It is not soluble in water and after early trials it was formulated in 'Cremophor EL'. It is now marketed as an emulsion in a soya bean oil/egg phosphatide and glycerol mixture. It is marketed in 20 ml vials (concentration 10 mg/ml) and unfortunately, once a vial is opened, any remaining unused at the end of day must be discarded since there in no bacteriocidal additive.

Pharmacology

i. The drug produces unconsciousness rapidly following I/V administration, although onset is slightly slower than that following thiopentone.

ii. Propofol is highly protein bound (98%) hence the active portion of any injected dose will be considerably enhanced in hypoproteinaemic states.

iii. Recovery from the effects of the drug depends on its rapid hepatic metabolism rather than on redistribution (elimination half-life is 30 minutes). The drug is therefore, non-cumulative and recovery is rapid with no 'hangover' effect.

iv. It produces a dose related degree of cardiovascular depression similar to the barbiturates. Therefore, hypotension tends to occur initially and occasionally a profound bradycardia may develop.

v. Respiratory depression also occurs in a dose related manner.

Use

Propofol is licensed for use in dogs and cats for the induction and maintenance of short term anaesthesia.

Although relatively expensive, propofol offers certain advantages over other short term anaesthetic agents which makes it the ideal choice in certain situations.

i. The rapid and full recovery of consciousness in some 15—20 minutes following a single I/V dose, means that this is a drug which can truly be used for day or post evening surgery cases. It is, therefore, ideal for the provision of restraint for radiography, suturing, grass seed removal etc.

ii. Its rapid metabolism also means that it can be used for the induction of anaesthesia for Caesarian Section. As long as the time interval between administration and foetal delivery is at least 10 minutes, the drug will have been metabolised by the dam allowing the foetuses to be delivered with minimal depression. The dam will recover quickly and will thus be able to nurse her offspring very quickly (see chapter 10).

Dog

Induction

Propofol alone:
5—6 mg/kg I/V (males appear to require a slightly higher dose compared to females).

In premedicated dogs:
3—4 mg/kg I/V.

Maintenance

An infusion of 0.4 mg/kg/min will maintain anaesthesia.

Recovery occurs within 18 minutes of the administration of a single dose.

Cats

Induction

6—7 mg/kg I/V. The dose does not appear to be influenced by prior sedation with acepromazine. A single dose produces anaesthesia lasting only approximately 10—15 minutes.

Maintenance:

An infusion rate of 0.51 mg/kg/min will maintain anaesthesia.

Recovery is rapid and occurs within 20—30 minutes following a single dose.

Some cats exhibit retching, sneezing and may paw their faces during recovery.

Problems:

i. Occasional transient profound bradycardia after I/V administration.

ii. Due to increased sensitivity in debilitated or old animals, the dose rate needs to be reduced considerably (2—3 mg/kg).

iii. Enhanced effect and prolonged duration of action is likely in animals suffering from liver dysfunction and/or hypoproteinaemia.

5. NEUROLEPTANAESTHETIC MIXTURES

Neuroleptanalgesic mixtures may be administered in order to provide sufficient depth of analgesia so that the animal becomes virtually unconscious. These drug combinations are only satisfactory for providing restraint and for allowing minor procedures to be carried out. They are insufficient, when used alone, to provide safe anaesthesia or reasonable operating conditions for major surgery. They are combinations of a potent opioid/narcotic and a sedative drug and are, therefore, used only in dogs.

Advantages

1. Ease of administration.
2. Potential for administration of an antagonist.

Disadvantages.

1. The narcotic component of these combinations produces such marked respiratory depression and cardiovascular impairment that it is essential to provide a secure airway and an oxygen enriched atmosphere if hypoxia is to be avoided.
2. The potent narcotic provides good analgesia but, unfortunately, the administration of the narcotic antagonist at the end of surgery not only reverses anaesthesia but abolishes all pain relief and renders the further administration of any narcotic analgesic useless.
3. Poor muscle relaxation.
4. These are controlled drugs under the Misuse of Drugs Act 1971.
5. Potential for accidental or deliberate self-administration, which may be fatal.
6. Sensitivity to noise and lights.
7. May cause defaecation and vomition.

Combinations available

a. **S.A. IMMOBILON,** (C Vet Ltd.)

   This combines etorphine 0.074 mg/ml and methotrimeprazine 18 mg/ml marketed together with **'Revivon'** (C Vet Ltd.) which contains diprenorphine 0.272 mg/ml.

   Dose:

   0.05 ml/kg I/V

   0.1 ml/kg I/M

   Onset:

   Immediately after I/V administration

   5 minutes after I/M administration

   Duration:

   60—90 minutes
   Full recovery will take up to 2 hours

   It is advisable to give atropine to counteract bradycardia.

   There is a **considerable degree of risk** associated with its use in elderly dogs and in debilitated or sick animals.

b. **HYPNORM** (Janssens)

This combines fluanisone 10 mg/ml and fentanyl 0.315 mg/ml.

Dose:

0.25 — 0.5 ml/kg

It is advisable to give atropine to counteract the bradycardia

Onset:

2 — 3 minutes

Duration:

30 minutes although fluanisone sedation lasts longer

Animals are very sensitive to noise

It is not recommended in debilitated, sick or elderly animals

CONCLUSIONS

The sole use of intravenous anaesthetic agents is only suitable for minor procedures of short duration.

For longer periods of surgery, a balanced technique should be employed, with intravenous induction of anaesthesia being followed by the maintenance of anaesthesia by inhalational means.

Despite appearing to offer the advantages of simplicity, the use of intravenous anaesthetic agents, without proper regard for normal, good anaesthetic management, cannot be condoned. It is always vital to ensure that the airway is open and secure from inhalation. Hypoventilation and hypoxia must be avoided and equipment for artificial ventilation with oxygen must be available. Lack of these basic facilities can no longer be defended.

In addition, proper care must be taken to ensure that hypothermia does not occur and that fluid balance is maintained and no animal should be discharged from the care of a veterinary surgeon until **fully recovered** from the effects of anaesthesia.

REFERENCES AND FURTHER READING

BREARLEY, J. C., KELLAGHER, R. E. B. and HALL, L. W. (1988). Propofol anaesthesia in cats. *J. small Anim. Pract.* **29**, 315-322.

CULLEN, L. K. and JONES, R. S. (1977). Clinical observations on xylazine/ketamine anaesthesia in the cat. *Vet. Rec.* **101**, 115-116.

GLENN, J. B. and HUNTER, S. C. (1984). The pharmacology of an emulsion formulation of ICI 35868. *Br. J. Anaesth.* **56**, 617-625.

HALL, L. W. and CHAMBERS, J. P. (1987). A clinical trial of propofol infusion anaesthesia in dogs. *J. small Anim. Pract.* **28**, 623-637.

HALL, L. W. and CLARKE, K. W. (1991). *Veterinary Anaesthesia.* 9th ed. Balliere Tindall.

HASKINS, S. C., PATZ, J. D. and FARVER, T. B. (1986). Xylazine and xylazine-ketamine in dogs. *Am. J. Vet. Res.* **47**, 636-641.

JONES, R. S. (1979). Injectable anaesthetic agents in the cats: a review. *J. small Anim. Pract.* **20**, 345-352.

WATKINS, S. B., HALL, L. W. and CLARKE, K. W. (1987). Propofol as an intravenous anaesthetic agent in dogs. *Vet. Rec.* **120**, 326-329.

YOUNG, L. E. and JONES, R. S. (1990). Clinical observations on medetomidine/ketamine anaesthesia and its antagonism by atipamezole in the cat. *J. small Animal. Pract.* **31**, 221-224.

CHAPTER 7

INHALATION ANAESTHESIA

R. S. Jones M.V.Sc., Dr. Med. Vet., D.V.Sc., D.V.A., F.I.Biol., F.R.C.V.S.

GASEOUS AND VOLATILE ANAESTHETIC AGENTS

Anaesthetic agents which are administered to animals by inhalation are either gases or volatile liquids. The only gas which is in common use is nitrous oxide. The commonly used liquids are diethyl ether, halothane, methoxyflurane, enflurane and isoflurane.

GAS

Nitrous Oxide

a. Physical Properties

Nitrous oxide is compressed to a pressure of 51 atmospheres in metal cylinders which are coloured blue. Two main impurities are produced during manufacture of the gas and must be removed before the gas is liquified. These are nitric oxide and nitrogen dioxide. The gas is in liquid form in the cylinder with a variable amount of free gas above the liquid. A reducing valve is essential. It is a sweet smelling, non-irritant, colourless gas and is heavier than air and is neither inflammable nor explosive but supports the combustion of other agents.

b. Pharmacological Properties

Nitrous oxide is rapidly eliminated unchanged from the body, mostly via the lungs. It is a potent analgesic but a weak anaesthetic and should, therefore, be administered in high concentrations. Care should be taken, however, to ensure that not less than 30% oxygen is administered with nitrous oxide. To avoid diffusion hypoxia at the end of a period of nitrous oxide administration, it is essential to administer 100% oxygen to the animal for at least 10 minutes before allowing it to breathe atmospheric air.

c. Uses

As nitrous oxide is a weak anaesthetic agent, it is difficult to maintain anaesthesia in animals with it as a sole agent. It should be administered after adequate premedication and an intravenous induction and supplemented with either a volatile or an intravenous agent. When muscle relaxants and intermittent positive pressure ventilation (IPPV) are employed, supplementation with other agents is also essential, but in lesser amounts than in the spontaneous breathing patient.

There are obvious advantages in the use of nitrous oxide and oxygen, rather than oxygen alone, in that the overall requirement for anaesthetic agents is reduced.

VOLATILE LIQUIDS

Diethyl Ether

a. Physical Properties

Diethyl ether is a colourless volatile liquid with a boiling point of 35°C and a vapour which is heavier than air. It is inflammable and explosive in oxygen. It is chemically relatively inert, but is decomposed by air, light and heat, and hence should be stored in dark bottles in a cool place.

b. Pharmacological Properties

Diethyl ether is largely unaltered in the body and the majority is eliminated by the lungs. The effects of ether on the heart and circulation are related to the depth of anaesthesia. Initially, the heart rate is stimulated due to the release of adrenaline and nor-adrenaline, but later the rate varies little from normal. A light plane of anaesthesia causes vasoconstriction and a deep one produces vasodilation. In deeper levels of anaesthesia, there is a progressive fall in blood pressure. Cardiac dysrhythmias are rare. Inhalation of ether stimulates the secretion of saliva and mucus. Respiratory movements are stimulated by ether vapour, although as anaesthesia deepens, the rate may increase, while the amplitude decreases. Nausea and vomiting occur in a high percentage of patients in the post-anaesthetic period. Muscular relaxation is excellent under ether anaesthesia, due to a direct neuromuscular block and to a reduction in motor nerve impulses.

c. Uses

Ether can be administered by any of the methods commonly employed for inhalation agents. It is, however, largely being superseded by newer products in veterinary anaesthesia, although there is probably still a place for its use in cats because of its relative safety. Since ether is explosive, its use is limited, but it can be administered satisfactorily in the dog by the semi-closed method as a supplement to oxygen or nitrous oxide and oxygen. Premedication with atropine is usually given to prevent excessive secretion of saliva and mucus and ether is added to the inhaled gases as early as possible during the administration and in increments of increasing concentration, so as to avoid coughing and breath-holding.

Halothane

a. Physical Properties

Halothane is a colourless volatile liquid with a boiling point of 50°C. It is non-inflammable and non-explosive when mixed in clinical concentrations with oxygen. It is decomposed by light and should be stored in amber coloured bottles.

b. Pharmacological Properties

Halothane is a potent anaesthetic agent and the vapour is pleasant to smell and non-irritant. Delivered concentrations of up to 4% are used for induction of anaesthesia and from 0.5% to 2% are used for maintenance. The arterial blood pressure falls during halothane anaesthesia and is proportional to the inhaled vapour concentration. The chief cause of the hypotension is probably a fall in cardiac output due to a depression of myocardial contractility. Dysrhythmias are not uncommon during halothane anaesthesia. Alimentary tract secretions are not stimulated. Halothane depresses respiration and often causes a decrease in alveolar ventilation. Muscular relaxation during halothane anaesthesia is only moderate, although it potentiates the duration of action of the non-depolarising, curare-type muscle relaxants such as alcuronium. Whilst a number of reports have appeared in the medical literature of 'halothane' hepatitis or 'halothane' jaundice in man, a considerable amount of controversy surrounds the subject. There is no real evidence to suggest that, under conditions of clinical anaesthesia, a similar condition occurs in animals. Whilst it was originally suggested that halothane was excreted unchanged by way of the lungs, experimental work has shown that this is not in fact the case, and up to 20% of halothane in the body may be degraded. Metabolites are slowly cleared from the body and may be present for as long as three weeks. Shivering and tremor are often seen in animals recovering from halothane anaesthesia, unrelated to temperature falls during anaesthesia.

c. Uses

Halothane can be administered by a number of different techniques, although, due to its potency and on economic grounds, it is best administered either in a semi-closed or a closed system (see Practical Administration of Inhalation Anaesthetics page 72).

Methoxyflurane

a. Physical Properties

Methoxyflurane is a halogen substituted methyl ethyl ether. It is a volatile liquid with a boiling point of 104°C and is non-inflammable and non-explosive and has a characteristic fruity odour.

b. Pharmacological Properties

Methoxyflurane is a good analgesic and produces good muscular relaxation. In deep anaesthesia, respirations are depressed and blood pressure falls. Dysrhythmias are uncommon. Most of the drug is excreted unchanged by way of the lungs but metabolism does occur. Metabolites are excreted in the urine over a long period of up to twelve days. In some species this may be important in the aetiology of renal toxicity.

c. Uses

As the induction of anaesthesia with methoxyflurane is slow due to its low volatility, it is wise to induce anaesthesia with an intravenous agent, after adequate premedication. It can be used in most types of anaesthetic circuits with either oxygen or nitrous oxide and oxygen. A comparison of methoxyflurane and halothane in small animal anaesthesia, has been made by Hall (1964).

Enflurane

a. Physical Properties

Enflurane is a halogen substituted ether. It is a volatile liquid with a boiling point of 56.5°C. Concentrations above 4.25% are inflammable in 20% oxygen in nitrous oxide. It is stable with soda-lime and metals. It contains no preservative.

b. Pharmacological Properties

Enflurane is a potent anaesthetic agent. It tends to produce EEG changes of an eleptiform nature, which are more common during hypocarbia and tend to persist for several weeks. As the depth of anaesthesia increases, there is a reversible fall in arterial blood pressure due to myocardial depression. Serious cardiac dysrhythmias are uncommon. Pulmonary ventilation is decreased; tidal volume is decreased with a variable rise in respiratory rate. It produces reasonable muscle relaxation and potentiates non-depolarising muscle relaxants. It is excreted mainly by the lungs but up to 2% of enflurane is metabolised in the body.

c. Uses

Enflurane is less potent than halothane so that a higher concentration is required for an equivalent effect. As it is more expensive than halothane, its use tends to be restricted to a closed circuit. Due to its relative insolubility, levels of anaesthesia can be changed rapidly whilst recovery is smooth and relatively rapid. Delivered concentrations of up to 5% are used for induction and 1.5–3% for maintenance.

Isoflurane

a. Physical Properties

Isoflurane is an isomer of enflurane. It is a colourless liquid with a similar saturated vapour pressure to that of halothane. Theoretically, it could be used in the same vaporiser as halothane, but this is not recommended on safety grounds. Induction of and recovery from anaesthesia are rapid partly due to its low blood/gas partition coefficient and partly due to its low fat solubility. Isoflurane is stable and no preservatives are necessary and it does not react with metal. It has a boiling point of 48.5°C.

b. Pharmacological Properties

Isoflurane is a myocardial depressant but its effects are less than enflurane or halothane. Arterial blood pressure falls during isoflurane anaesthesia, due mainly to a fall in systemic vascular resistance. Isoflurane anaesthesia produces stable cardiac rhythm, but the rate may be increased. It tends to produce a decrease in tidal volume and an increase in respiratory rate. It does not produce changes in the EEG. About 0.2% of inhaled isoflurane is metabolised.

c. Uses

The high cost of isoflurane tends to limit its use in veterinary anaesthesia. However, where it is used, it tends to be used in closed circuits. It provides stability of cardiac rhythm and does not sensitise the heart to adrenaline. Hence, there are specific indications for its use in various cardiac conditions, such as traumatic myocarditis. As it is a stable molecule, it is unlikely to produce organ toxicity. Delivered concentrations of up to 4% isoflurane may be used for induction of anaesthesia and 1.5 to 2% for maintenance. The use of isoflurane in dogs has been described by Jones and Seymour (1986).

GASES USED IN ASSOCIATION WITH ANAESTHESIA

Oxygen

Oxygen is prepared by the fractional distillation of liquid air and is supplied in cylinders at a pressure of 135 atmospheres. The cylinders are available in a number of sizes. In contact with oil or grease, oxygen under pressure will cause a fire but is not itself inflammable.

Carbon Dioxide

Carbon dioxide is a colourless non-inflammable gas which is rapidly absorbed from the alveoli. It is prepared by the action of heat on carbonates and is stored in grey-coloured cylinders after compression to 50 atmospheres. It has a number of uses in anaesthesia, the main ones being:-

i. to increase the depth of anaesthesia when volatile agents are used and hence increase the speed of induction.

ii. to stimulate the onset of respiration after a period of intermittent positive pressure ventilation. It is not advisable to use the gas to stimulate respiration during resuscitation.

BASIC TECHNIQUES FOR ADMINISTRATION OF INHALATION AGENTS

Inhalation agents may be administered by one of four techniques.

1. The Open Method

The open method, which is rarely used nowadays but may be utilised in an emergency if other equipment is not available, involves placing some absorbent material near to the animal's face and dropping the anaesthetic agent onto it. The depth of anaesthesia cannot be controlled accurately but depends on the rate at which the agent is dropped onto the material. With this technique, hypoxia and hypercapnia are likely to develop and effective resuscitation is difficult.

2. The Semi-Open Method

The semi-open method involves the use of absorbent material in a mask, through which the air is inhaled. The technique has similar disadvantages to the open method.

3. The Semi-Closed Method

The semi-closed method involves the use of an anaesthetic machine and an anaesthetic circuit. Most of the commonly used semi-closed circuits do not incorporate carbon dioxide absorption. The fresh gas flow must, therefore, be used to eliminate carbon dioxide from the circuit. A theoretical study of various semi-closed circuits has been carried out by Mapleson (1954). In veterinary anaesthesia, two main types of semi-closed circuit are in use, but two other types have also been described and used to a lesser extent.

They are:

a. The Magill Circuit (Mapleson A).

This consists of a reservoir bag, wide corrugated tube, an expiratory valve (Heidebrink) and a connector to either a mask or endotracheal tube. During inspiration, anaesthetic gases are inhaled from the reservoir bag; on expiration, the exhaled gases pass out to the atmosphere by way of the expiratory valve and also pass back up the corrugated tubing. During the expiratory pause, before the next inspiration, the flow of gas from the machine forces the rest of the expired gases out to the atmosphere through the expiratory valve. It is important to note that for effective operation, a flow rate at least equal to, and preferably greater than, the animal's minute volume, is required to ensure adequate removal of carbon dioxide from the circuit.

In practice, there is no upper weight of animal for which this type of circuit can be used, but at higher weights the flow rates required may prove uneconomical. The Magill circuit can be used on animals with weights as low as 5 kg. A typical circuit is shown in Figures 7.1 and 7.2.

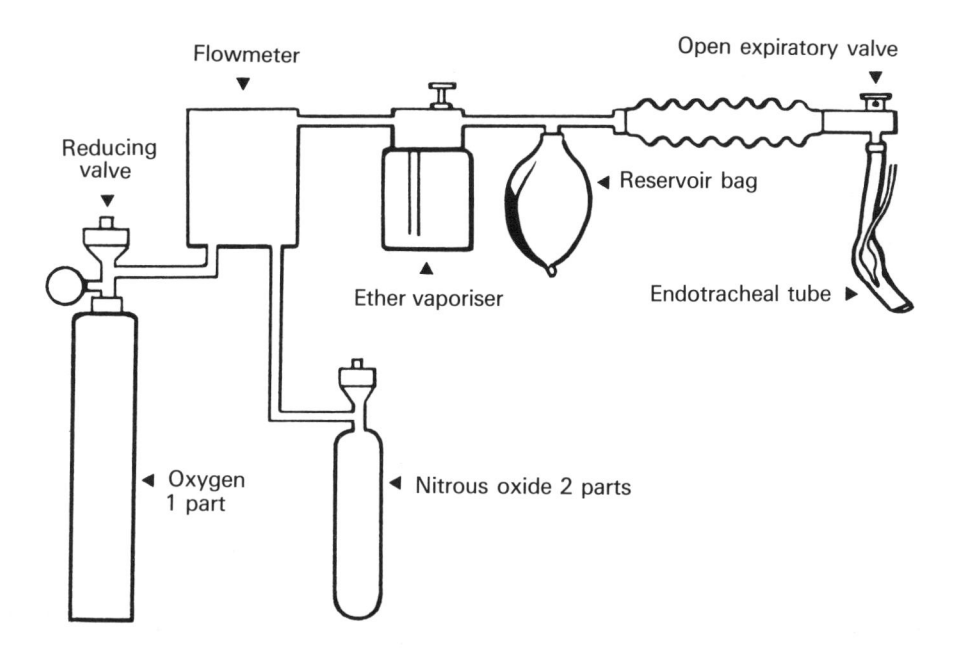

Figure 7.1
The apparatus for administering nitrous oxide/oxygen and a volatile agent in semi-closed circuit by endotracheal tube.

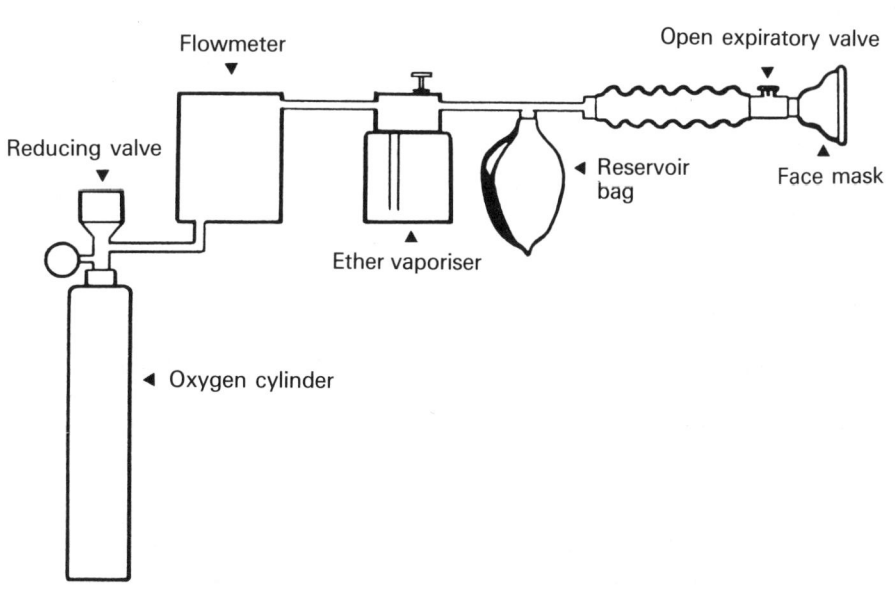

Figure 7.2
The apparatus for administering oxygen and ether in a semi-closed circuit with a mask.

b. The Ayre's T-piece (Mapleson E)
This is recommended for use in small dogs and cats up to 5 kg weight. It has no valves and hence there is very little resistance to breathing. A typical Ayre's T-piece with an open-ended bag mounted on the expiratory limb, is shown in Figure 7.3.

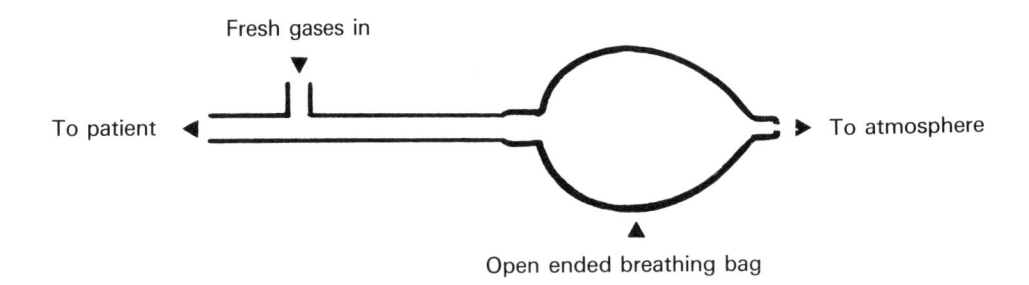

Figure 7.3

A Jackson-Rees modification of an Ayre's T-piece.

c. The Bain Co-axial Circuit (Mapleson D)
The use of the Bain circuit in veterinary anaesthesia has been described by Carlucci and Hird (1978). There are no valves and hence the circuit produces very little resistance to breathing. As the expiratory port is near the anaesthetic machine, it is particularly useful for surgery of the head and neck.

d. The Lack System (Mapleson A)
This is a modification of the Magill system. The patient breathes through both tubes. The outer tube is inspiratory and the inner is expiratory with the valve situated near the anaesthetic apparatus. The inspiratory limb has a capacity of 500 ml but does not readily permit the use of mechanical ventilators. The Lack system is superior in performance to both the Bain and Magill circuits, as it is relatively economical in the use of fresh gas and has an accessible exhaust valve. Its use in veterinary anaesthesia has been described by Waterman (1986).

Non-rebreathing Valves

A number of non-rebreathing valves have been used in anaesthesia, particularly with the Magill circuit. They prevent a build-up of carbon dioxide and can be used to measure minute volume since the amount of gas exhaled is equal to that being delivered from the flow meters. Nevertheless, the valves can stick and are wasteful of expensive agents. The only one that has been used to any extent is the Ruben's valve.

4. The Closed Method

This requires an anaesthetic machine and an anaesthetic circuit. The anaesthetic system incorporates soda lime to absorb the exhaled dioxide. Since high flow rates are not required to remove the carbon dioxide, it is an economical method of administering inhalation anaesthetic agents. It should be noted that the closed method should not be used in cats or dogs under 10 kg weight due to the resistance to respiration provided by the soda lime.

When this method is used, the anaesthetic agent plus oxygen, is inhaled by the animal and the mixture is exhaled, less some oxygen and plus some carbon dioxide. If the mixture is passed through soda lime to remove carbon dioxide and into a reservoir bag, it can be rebreathed. Therefore, only small amounts of oxygen are required to meet the animal's metabolic requirements. Whilst theoretically, more anaesthetic agent is not required, it has to be added to compensate for leaks, passage into rubber and uptake by the body.

Soda lime consists of 90% calcium hydroxide, 5% sodium hydroxide and 1% potassium hydroxide with silicates to prevent powdering. It is essential for effective absorption, that moisture be incorporated within the granule. The hydroxides combine with carbon dioxide in the presence of water to form carbonates.

The advantages of a closed circuit are economy in the use of gases and less risk of explosion. Heat and moisture are conserved and there is less pollution of the atmosphere. The disadvantages are that soda lime produces resistance to breathing and alkaline dust may be inhaled by the patient.

In veterinary anaesthesia, two types of closed circuit apparatus are employed:-

a. The 'To-and-Fro' System

This is by far the commonest one in general use, consisting of an endotracheal tube (occasionally a mask), a connector, separated from the re-breathing bag by a Water's canister of soda lime (Figure 7.4). Gases pass through the canister both on inspiration and expiration. The original canister was designed for medical use and is of critical size. However, with the variations in the size of dogs, it is difficult to choose a canister which has an air space approximately equal to the animal's tidal volume. In practice, provided the animal is over 10 kg in weight, it does not appear to be of great importance.

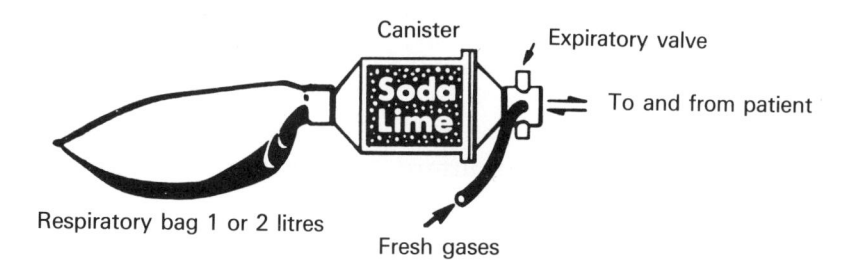

Figure 7.4
To and fro closed circuit (Water's canister).

b. The Circle System

This is more complex and hence more expensive than the to-and-fro closed system. The inspiratory and expiratory tubes are used with one-way valves to produce an unidirectional flow of gases within the system. A soda lime canister and a rebreathing bag are incorporated into the circuit and occasionally a vaporiser as well. In most closed circuit systems, it is possible to by-pass the soda lime canister and hence it can be easily removed for refilling during an anaesthetic. Closed circuit circle systems (Figure 7.5) are very efficient in the removal of carbon dioxide, but due to the valves and long tubing, have a higher resistance to respiration than the to-and-fro system.

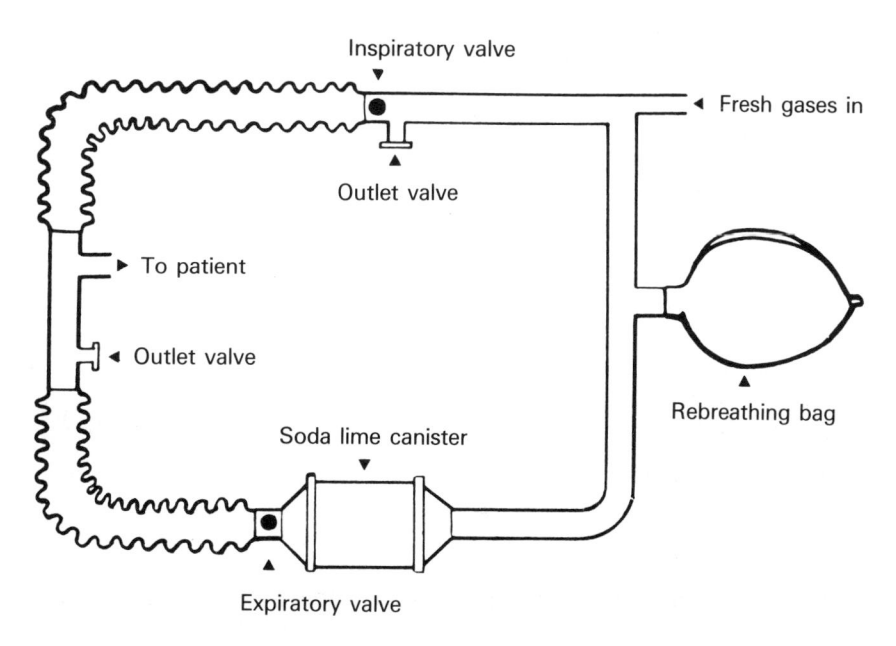

Figure 7.5
Closed circuit circle absorber system.

FLOW RATES

The tidal volume is the volume of air inspired or expired in a single breath. The minute volume is the volume of air inspired or expired in one minute. Hence the minute volume is obtained by multiplying the tidal volume by the respiratory rate. In the normal dog and cat, the tidal volume is between 10 and 15 ml/kg. The lower weight animals tend to have the higher value. An arbitrary value of 20 breaths per minute is usually quoted for the respiratory rate. However, smaller animals tend to have a higher frequency of up to 30 per minute and larger animals have a lower frequency which can be as low as 15 per minute. Hence, using the value for tidal volume and counting the respiratory rate, it is possible to calculate the minute volume. In Bain and Ayres 'T'piece circuits, a flow rate of 2½ – 3 times the minute volume is required. The Magill and Lack circuits only require a flow rate equal to the minute volume. The oxygen consumption of the average dog and cat is 4 – 5 ml/kg/min. and hence this is the theoretical minimum required for use in a closed circuit. However, due to inefficiency of all common anaesthetic vaporisers and the likelihood of nitrogen build up in a closed circuit, a minimum flow rate of 1 litre of oxygen per minute is advisable.

ARTIFICIAL VENTILATION (Intermittent Positive Pressure Ventilation or I.P.P.V.)

Uses and effects.

Artificial ventilation may be used under a number of different circumstances during anaesthesia. The most obvious one is during the resuscitation of apnoeic patients. It is also used during intrathoracic surgery. In addition, it is also necessary when muscle relaxants are used as part of an anaesthetic technique for surgery of parts of the body other than the thorax.

During intermittent positive pressure ventilation, a number of physiological changes occur. Inspiratory, intrapulmonary and intrapleural pressures are the reverse of what is found in normal breathing i.e. they are positive instead of negative. One of the most important effects produced by I.P.P.V. is on the venous return to the heart. The right atrial pressure is raised and venous return and cardiac output are reduced. This is usually compensated for by a rise in peripheral venous pressure brought about by venoconstriction. Where venoconstriction is maximal, as in hypovolaemic shock, harmful effects can be seen. Therefore, before using I.P.P.V., it is essential to ensure that the blood volume is within normal limits. Mean intrathoracic pressure can be reduced by shortening the duration of inspiration and hence allowing more time between inspirations (longer expiratory pause), and by introducing a negative pressure in the expiratory phase which should not exceed -5cm, H_2O.

PRACTICAL ADMINISTRATION OF INHALATION ANAESTHETICS

Whilst it is not desirable, or even possible in a manual of this nature, to discuss the practical administration of all agents in both the dog and cat, it is reasonable to offer guidelines for at least one agent that is used in both species. Halothane is the best choice for this since it is in widespread use and is considered relatively safe. With an adequate knowledge of the pharmacology of other drugs and the correct equipment, information on the techniques for using one drug can then be readily transposed to another.

Practical Administration of Halothane

1. First, check the anaesthetic machine, noting the state of the cylinders and vaporiser and taking care to ensure that adequate amounts of gas and anaesthetic agent are available for the particular procedure to be carried out.

2. Select a suitable circuit and attach it to the anaesthetic machine. For dogs, depending on the body size and procedure being undertaken, either a semi-closed or a closed circuit; for cats a semi-closed circuit — an Ayre's T-piece.

3. Premedicate with atropine or glycopyrrolate (optional) and acepromazine (See Chapter 5).

4. Induce anaesthesia with either

    a. thiopentone using a syringe containing dose of 1 ml of a 2.5% solution per kg and, under normal circumstances, administering half the dose by rapid intravenous injection (N.B. in cats use a 1.25% solution of thiopentone instead of a 2.5% solution and see Chapter 6);

    b. oxygen or preferably oxygen and nitrous oxide and halothane (4 – 6%) administered from a semi-closed circuit by mask.

5. In the dog: once the animal is relaxed, open the jaws and intubate with an endotracheal tube, inflate the cuff and connect the tube to the circuit of choice; face masks can be used but are rarely preferred. In the cat: face masks are commonly used in preference to intubation. If endotracheal intubation is to be performed, a muscle relaxant must be given or the larynx sprayed with lignocaine to produce suitable conditions before passing the tube.

6. After induction and intubation, give a relatively high concentration of halothane (4%) with either oxygen or nitrous oxide and oxygen, depending on the type of circuit; nitrous oxide is only used with a semi-closed circuit and not less than 30% oxygen should be administered with it.

7. Take care to ensure that spontaneous ventilation starts in a relatively short time. If not, switch off halothane, empty the reservoir bag and refill with oxygen; inflate the lungs by rhythmical compression of the reservoir bag.

8. Place a finger on the femoral pulse, note changes and act on them; or, preferably, pass an oesophageal stethoscope as soon after endotracheal intubation as possible and monitor pulse rate with this.

9. Once the palpebral reflex has disappeared and respiration settles to a steady state (the rate of respiration can vary from animal to animal), reduce the concentration of halothane to 2%, 1.5% or even 1%, depending on the response of the animal to surgery. When anaesthesia is induced with halothane and a mask, the concentration is adjusted in a similar manner.

10. Observe the animal closely throughout the period of anaesthesia, noting pulse and respiratory rate at 5 minute intervals. Note any response of the patient; observe the colour and refill time of visible mucous membranes. The percentage of halothane should be increased in response to any changes in the respiratory rate and any movement on the part of the animal. It is rarely necessary to exceed 4% halothane.

11. At the end of the surgical procedure, if nitrous oxide has been used, it should be switched off and the oxygen flow increased to maintain the same total flow rate for at least 10 minutes before the animal is allowed to breathe room air. Halothane can be switched off once the closure of the skin incision has started.

12. Once surgery has been completed, the animal is allowed to breathe room air, placed in a recovery area and observed closely. When the animal starts to cough or gag on the endotracheal tube, it is removed and the tongue pulled forward out of the mouth. Check to ensure that the airway remains clear and keep the animal warm during the recovery period.

REFERENCES

HALL, L. W. (1964) A comparison of methoxyflurane and halothane in small animal anaesthesia. *Vet. Rec.* **76**, 650.

HIRD, J. F. R. and CARLUCCI, F. (1978) A new anaesthetic circuit for use in the dog. *J. small Anim. Pract.* **19**, 277.

JONES, R. S. and SEYMOUR, C. J. (1986) Clinical experience with isoflurane in dogs and horses. *Vet. Rec.* **119**, 8-10.

MAPLESON, W. W. (1954) The elimination of rebreathing in various semi-closed anaesthetic systems. *Brit. J. Anaesth.* **26**, 323.

WATERMAN, A. E. (1986) Evaluation of the Lack breathing in small animal anaesthesia. *J. small Anim. Pract.* **27.**, 591-598.

FURTHER READING

HALL, L. W. and CLARKE, K. W. (1991) Veterinary Anaesthesia 9th ed. Balliere, Tindall.
LUMB, W. V. and JONES, E. W. (1984) Veterinary Anaesthesia, 2nd ed. Lea and Febiger, Philadelphia.

CHAPTER 8

LOCAL ANAESTHESIA

K. W. Clarke M.A., Vet. MB., D.Vet.Med., D.V.A., M.R.C.V.S.

GENERAL CONSIDERATIONS

Local anaesthetic solutions may be used in the following ways to produce analgesia.

1.	SURFACE	e.g.: Mucous membranes Cornea Intrasynovial analgesia.
2.	LOCAL INFILTRATION	e.g.: Directly at surgical site Field Blocks
3.	REGIONAL	e.g.: Specific nerve blocks Spinal analgesia Epidural analgesia
4.	INTRAVENOUS REGIONAL ANALGESIA	e.g.: Limbs

Although regional techniques are rarely used in Britain in small animals because of the ease and comparative safety of general anaesthesia, they are, nevertheless, completely applicable. Full details of the many regional blocks possible are beyond the scope of this book and those seeking further details should refer to anatomy books and to the references mentioned at the end of this chapter.

USE OF ADRENALINE WITH LOCAL ANAESTHETICS

Most local analgesic drugs (except cocaine) cause vasodilation and the resultant increase in blood supply, both limits the action of the analgesic and increases systemic toxicity by increasing the speed of absorption. Adrenaline, through its vasoconstrictor activity, will counteract this effect. Preparations may be purchased containing adrenaline, but, as under some conditions of storage, its activity decreases, it may, if required, be added at the time of use. A concentration of 1 in 200,000 is adequate (a needle hub filled with 1 in 1000 adrenaline for 10 to 20 ccs of lignocaine is a suitable approximation).

Warning.

The vasoconstriction produced by adrenaline may cause ischaemic damage. Thus, hair may change colour after intradermal or subcutaneous administration and ring blocks around areas of limited blood supply, such as the teats of mammary glands, may cause necrosis.

LOCAL ANALGESIC DRUGS

Cocaine was the first local analgesic drug used. Despite its good analgesic properties, its high toxicity and the fact that it causes addiction in man (it is a controlled drug), mean that it is rarely used in veterinary practice. Several local analgesic agents, differing in length of action, rate of absorption, spread within the tissue, local irritability and toxicity, are marketed.

Those most commonly used in veterinary practice include:-

1. **Lignocaine,** synonym Lidocaine, 'Xylocaine', (Astra). (Many other commercial preparations available).
   This effective and versatile drug is suitable for use in almost all circumstances requiring a local analgesic agent.

   Its properties include:-

   a. excellent surface analgesia.

   b. effective spread throughout the tissue.

   c. minimal tissue irritation.

   d. rapid onset of action.

   e. action of about 1 hour (1 ½ hours with adrenaline).

   f. low toxicity.

   g. anti-arrhythmic action on the heart.

   h. stability on autoclaving.

   Systemic toxicity.

   The first signs of overdosage are drowsiness and sedation (N.B. lignocaine is the only commonly used local analgesic to show this phase). Further dosage results in twitching, convulsions and eventually coma and death. The actual dose required to cause these symptoms will obviously be influenced by the site of use and speed of absorption. The maximum recommended dose of lignocaine by infiltration to a medium sized dog is 0.6 grammes (30 mls of a 2% solution injection).

   Preparations of Lignocaine available include:-

   a. Solutions for injection of concentrations from 0.5% to 3%. Multidose bottles, single dose bottles and vials of various sizes are available, and most can be obtained with or without adrenaline.

   N.B. Some multidose preparations contain preservatives.

   b. Cartridges for use in a dental syringe, with or without adrenaline.

   c. Aerosol spray for surface analgesia.

   d. Gel, for lubrication with analgesia.

   e. Creams and ointments.

   f. Ophthalmic preparations.

2. **Procaine,** (many commercial preparations available).

   Procaine is still widely used in veterinary practice. Concentrations of between 1% and 5% have been employed, with or without the use of vasoconstrictors. It provides good analgesia for about an hour. However, it is a very poor surface analgesic and has weak powers of tissue penetration so that techniques of regional nerve blocks using this drug must be more accurate than if lignocaine is employed. Symptoms of procaine toxicity include twitching and convulsions followed by coma. However, the drug is rapidly broken down by liver enzymes and cumulative toxicity is therefore rare.

   N.B. Procaine should not be used in animals receiving sulphonamide treatment as the break down products of the analgesic (para-aminobenzoic acid) antagonises the effects of the sulphonamide drugs.

3. **Prilocaine,** 'Citanest', (Astra).

    Onset of analgesia is slower with this drug, due to less effective spreading properties. It does, however, cause minimal local irritation.

4. **Amethocaine.**

    A member of the procaine series, amethocaine is a powerful surface analgesic and is incorporated in many skin and aural preparations.

5. **Bupivacaine,** 'Marcaine', (Duncan Flockhart).

    Bupivacaine has a longer action than lignocaine and may be useful when prolonged analgesia is required.

6. **Proparacaine,** 'Opthaine V', (Squibb).

    Used as an opthalmic preparation.

SOME LOCAL ANAESTHETIC TECHNIQUES

1. **INTRAVENOUS REGIONAL ANALGESIA OF THE LIMBS**

    Uses

    This technique gives excellent analgesia of the lower limbs and is useful for any surgery of this region, such as amputation of digits, removal of inter-digital foreign bodies, etc.

    The technique is very simple and is carried out as follows:-

    1. The patient is restrained on its side (with or without sedation as found necessary.)
    2. An intravenous catheter or needle is placed in a suitable distal vein.
    3. The limb is partially exsanguinated either by use of an Esmarch's bandage or, less effectively but still adequately, by holding the limb up for 2 minutes.
    4. A tourniquet, which must be tight enough to stop arterial flow, is placed around the limb at a suitable point, proximal to the surgical site.
    5. 1% lignocaine WITHOUT ADRENALINE (2—3 ml is a suitable dose for a greyhound), is injected through the previously implanted catheter.

    Within 5—10 minutes, intense analgesia develops below the tourniquet and remains as long as the tourniquet is in position. At the end of the procedure, when the tourniquet is removed, the dog should still be restrained on its side for a few minutes.

    The main reasons for failure are an inadequate tourniquet, or failure to give sufficient time for analgesia to develop.

    Dangers include:-

    a. Inadvertent injection into the main bloodstream (i.e tourniquet not even stopping venous flow).
    b. Ischaemic damage from the tourniquet.
    c. Ischaemic pain and hypotension on removal of the tourniquet.

    With practice, this is a very simple and effective technique.

2. AURICULO-PALPEBRAL BLOCK

Uses

This branch of the facial nerve is the motor nerve to the orbicularis muscle and block, therefore, gives no analgesia but paralyses the eyelids. Uses include facilitation of examination of the eye; abolition of the palpebral reflex (which can be useful during surgery of the eyelids in cases which will not tolerate deep anaesthesia) and following intra-ocular surgery to reduce excessive blinking in the post operative period.

Technique

1 ml of 1% or 2% lignocaine is injected through skin and fascia, the site being at the upper border of the posterior part of the zygomatic arch, where the arch turns inwards (see Figure 8.1).

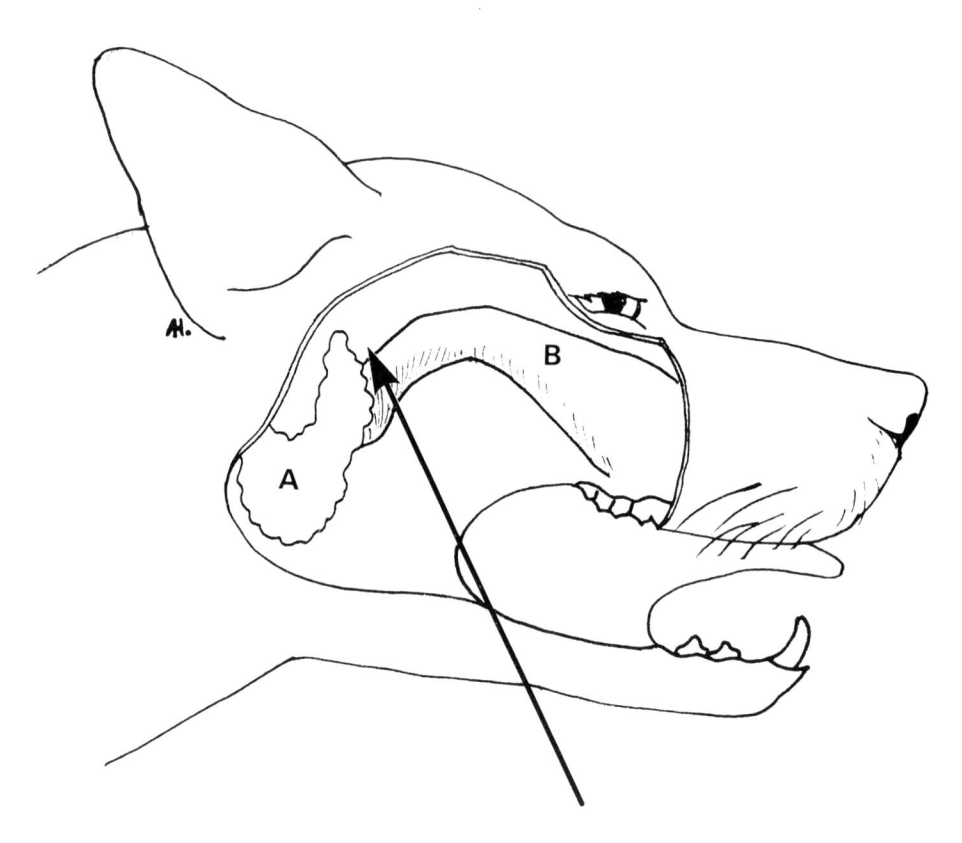

Figure 8.1
Auriculopalpebral block in the dog.

A. Parotid salivary gland.   B. Zygomatic arch.

3. LUMBAR EPIDURAL ANALGESIA

In the dog, with practice, lumbar epidural analgesia can be a reasonably safe and simple method of obtaining analgesia of the abdominal, caudal and hindquarter regions. The technique consists of injection of local analgesic solution into the epidural space at the lumbosacral junction. The solution spreads both anteriorly and posteriorly; the degree and direction of spread depending on the volume and concentration of the solution and the direction of the bevel of the needle. The spinal cord in the dog terminates at the sixth or seventh lumbar vertebrae and, although the meningeal sac continues into the sacral region, it is very small and inadvertent subarachnoid puncture is unlikely. (See Figure 8.2).

The technique may also be used in the cat, although problems of restraint make it of less use in this species.

a. Uses and Advantages

The technique may be used for any laparotomy, for hind limb analgesia or for analgesia of the perineal region. However, it is particularly useful for laparotomy in the very toxic animal, or for caesarian section. In both cases it gives excellent analgesia and muscle relaxation, yet avoids the need for general anaesthesia.

Complications:

a. Infection. Aseptic precautions MUST be taken throughout.

b. Hypotension. This occurs through interference with autonomic nerves. An intravenous infusion should be set up at the start of the procedure and vasopressor agents be available.

c. Systemic toxicity, through inadvertent I/V injection or rapid absorption from the epidural space.

d. Respiratory paralysis, if the block goes anteriorly to the cervical region.

e. Subarachnoid puncture, rare.

f. Spinal cord damage due to direct puncture (rare) or haemorrhage.

g. Failure of analgesia through faulty technique.

h. Hypothermia, particularly in small dogs and cats.

Emergency equipment which should also be available, includes:-

Intravenous fluids

Oxygen

Mechanism for artificial ventilation (including endotracheal tubes)

Vasopressors

b. Preparation of the patient

An intravenous infusion should be set up in order to maintain an 'open vein'. Premedication or sedation may be given if required. The lumbosacral region should be clipped and cleaned.

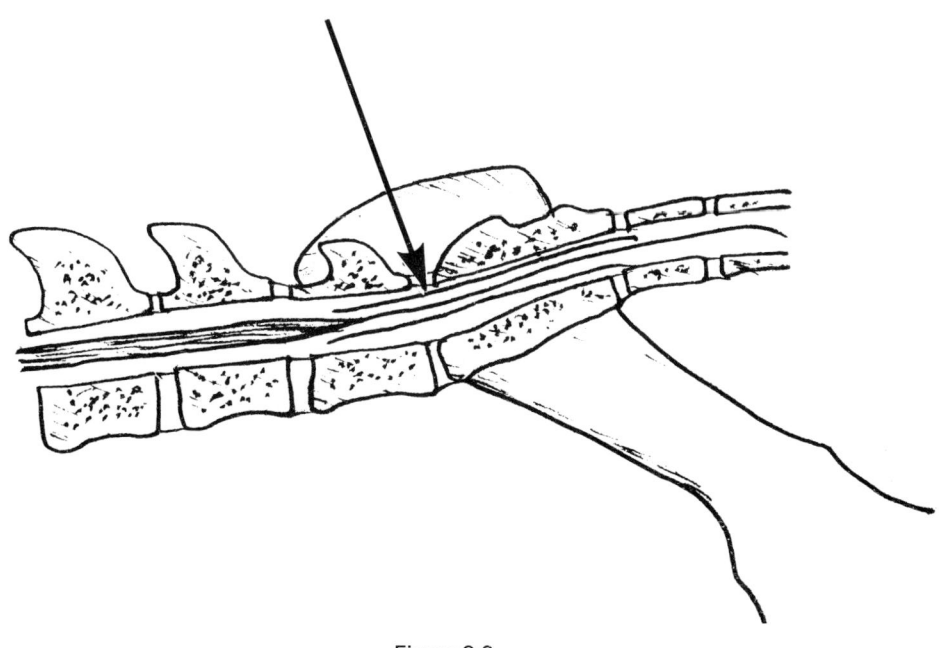

Figure 8.2
Epidural space in the dog

c. **Location of site** (see Figure 8.3).

The cranial dorsal iliac spines of the ileum can be palpated. The lumbosacral space is situated caudal to a line drawn between these and is just posterior to the spinous process of the seventh lumbar vertebra.

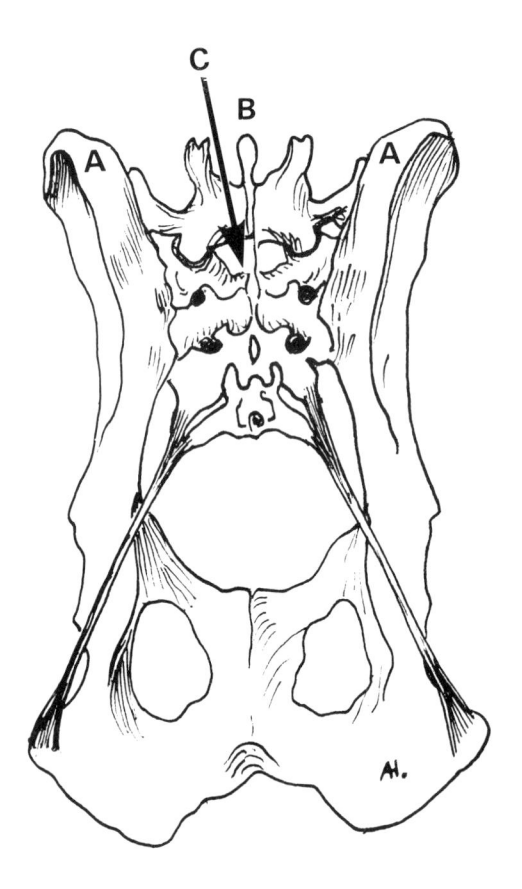

Figure 8.3
Lumbosacral space in the dog.
A: Cranial Dorsal iliac spines.
B: Spinous process L7.
C: Lumbosacral intervertebral space.

Injection Technique.

N.B. ASEPTIC TECHNIQUE ESSENTIAL

The patient is restrained either on its side or in the sternal position supported by an assistant. The former method has the advantage of reducing the chance of sudden movements. The site is located, cleaned and the anaesthetist (wearing sterile gloves), infiltrates the skin and muscle with 2% lignocaine. The epidural needle is introduced directly in the midline, either perpendicular to the skin or pointing slightly backwards (Figure 8.3). Successful penetration of the interarcuate ligament usually results in a 'popping' sensation. Should the needle strike bone, it should be withdrawn slightly, then redirected either slightly forward, backward or to one side. Once thought to be in place, the needle should be aspirated to check that no blood or cerebrospinal fluid (CSF) can be aspirated. N.B. CSF may flow slowly from this site, so sufficient time must be given for this test. There should be no resistance to a test injection of air or local anaesthetic.

Once satisfied that the needle is in the epidural space, the required volume of local anaesthetic is injected slowly (10–15 seconds). Rapid injection leads to a patchy block and can cause discomfort, vomiting and convulsions.

The position of the patient may, at this stage, be altered to assist the spread of the analgesic. For example, a head down position helps the solution to spread forward, or a lateral position may lead to a unilateral block.

Analgesic and Dose.

Although many analgesics can be used, a 1% solution of lignocaine is very satisfactory.

The dose required depends on the size of the patient and the degree of block required. For most laparotomies, it is necessary to block to T5 and for this, doses of from 1.5 ml for a small dog, up to 11 mls for a large dog, have been recommended. A dose of 11 mls should only be exceeded with care. These dose rates give about 45 minutes of analgesia, which is lengthened to 1 ½ hours if 1 in 200,000 adrenaline is added to the solution. However, the degree and duration of block produced by a standard dose show great variations between individual animals.

Continuous epidural.

If a longer period of analgesia is required, further doses of about half the original volume of analgesia may be given as required. This is made easier if, in the first place, a plastic catheter is placed via a Touhy needle, into the epidural space.

FURTHER READING

EVANS, H. E. and CHRISTENSEN, G. C. *Miller's Anatomy of the Dog.* (1979) 2nd ed. W. B. Saunders.
HALL, L. W. and CLARKE, K. W. (1991). *Veterinary Anaesthesia.* 9th ed. Balliere, Tindall.
SOMA, L. R. (1971) *A Textbook of Veterinary Anaesthesia.* Baltimore, Williams and Wilkins.
TUFVESSON, G. *Local Anaesthesia in Veterinary Medicine.* Astra International Division of A. B. Astra, Soderlage, Sweden.
WILKINS, M. and FRITSCH, R. *Animal Anaesthesia Vol. 1: Local Anaesthesia.* Oliver and Boyd.

CHAPTER 9

USE OF MUSCLE RELAXANTS

G. J. Brouwer B.Vet.Med., B.Sc., D.V.A., M.R.C.V.S.

GENERAL CONSIDERATIONS

Neuromuscular blocking agents (muscle relaxants) produce muscle relaxation but have no analgesic or anaesthetic effect. They are used as part of a balanced anaesthetic protocol which should ensure that the patient is unconscious throughout. Under muscle relaxants it is more difficult to assess the depth of anaesthesia; good experience with non-relaxant anaesthetic techniques and a sound knowledge of the pharmacology of the anaesthetic agents being used concurrently, is highly desirable before using muscle relaxants for the first time. Paralysis of the respiratory muscles means that intermittent positive pressure ventilation (IPPV) needs to be applied; a thorough understanding of the equipment used to administer IPPV is essential.

INDICATIONS

1. To relax skeletal muscles for easier surgical access (especially laparotomy).
2. To facilitate control of respiration during thoracic surgery.
3. To assist reduction of dislocated joints.
4. To facilitate atraumatic endotracheal intubation in cats, and endoscopy in all animals.
5. To permit reduction in the amount of general anaesthetic used when muscle relaxation is not the prime requirement.

CONTRAINDICATIONS

1. Absence of adequate facilities for IPPV.
2. Doubts about the ability to assess the level of consciousness.

Relaxants should be used with great care in animals suffering from hypovolaemia, electrolyte imbalances or myasthenia.

TECHNIQUE OF USE

The precise technique will vary with personal preference. Premedication should include an anticholinergic since some relaxants cause marked salivation and also to counter the muscarinic effects (salivation and bradycardia) produced by neostigmine when used to reverse neuromuscular blockade. Venous access throughout the anaesthetic will be required and cannulation of at least one peripheral vein is to be recommended.

Anaesthesia is usually induced intravenously (e.g. thiopentone or propofol) followed by endotracheal intubation. Intubation is essential to secure a patient's airway, to prevent aspiration of gastric reflux via a relaxed oesophagus and to prevent inflation of the stomach when IPPV is applied to the upper airway.

IPPV is applied via an appropriate anaesthetic circuit or ventilator using oxygen alone (when anaesthesia is maintained intravenously) or using oxygen with nitrous oxide supplemented with low concentrations of volatile anaesthetic (e.g. 0.5% halothane or 0.2% methoxyflurane).

The muscle relaxant is given by **slow** intravenous injection; initial doses are shown below and these can be supplemented with half dose increments when necessary. Depolarising and non-depolarising muscle relaxants should not be mixed.

NEUROMUSCULAR BLOCKING DRUGS

Depolarising muscle relaxants

1. **Suxamethonium** 'Anectine' (Wellcome)
   Cat: 2-5 mg total dose; duration, 5 minutes.
   Dog: 0.3 mg/kg; duration 10-20 minutes. Suxamethonium is rarely helpful for anything other than minor procedures since topping-up can lead to prolonged blockade (dual-block).

Non-depolarising (competitive) muscle relaxants

1. **Pancuronium,** 'Pavulon' (Organon Teknika).
   Cat and Dog: 0.06—0.1 mg/kg; duration, 20—40 minutes.
   A generally safe and useful agent.
2. **Gallamine,** 'Flaxedil' (Rhone-Poulenc Rorer).
   Cat and Dog: 1—2 mg/kg; duration, 15—30 minutes. Renal insufficiency is a specific contraindication to the use of this drug.
3. **Alcuronium,** 'Alloferin' (Roche).
   Cat and Dog: 0.1 mg/kg; duration 15—30 minutes. Characterised by a slow onset of action. Repeated doses can lead to a persistent blockade difficult to reverse.
4. **Vercuronium,** 'Norcuron' (Organon Teknika).
   Dog: 0.05—0.1 mg/kg; duration 20—30 minutes. Very similar to pancuronium. Post-operative nausea and vomiting occasionally noted.
5. **Atracurium,** 'Tracrium' (Wellcome).
   Dog: 0.3—0.5 mg/kg; duration 20—30 minutes. Repeated doses do not show a cumulative trend. It is readily reversed and is the relaxant of choice in myasthenic patients.

The duration of action of any muscle relaxant can be potentiated by the concurrent use of volatile anaesthetic agents, certain antibiotics (e.g. neomycin and streptomycin) and organophosphorus compounds (e.g. insecticides and flea collars). Few, if any, of these muscle relaxants will be specifically licensed for use in animals.

SIGNS OF AWAKENING UNDER MUSCLE RELAXANTS

1. Increase in pulse rate not related to haemorrhage.
2. Signs of vasovagal syncope (hypotension, pallor).
3. Increase in end-tidal carbon dioxide gas tension, unrelated to IPPV pattern changes.
4. Lacrymation and increased salivation.
5. Occurrence of slight muscle movement (of the face, limbs or tongue) in response to stimulation.

It is essential that the patient remains fully unconscious whilst under the influence of muscle relaxants. Eye reflexes and movement are blocked by muscle relaxants and cannot be used to assess depth of anaesthesia reliably.

REVERSAL OF NEUROMUSCULAR BLOCKADE

Depolarising muscle relaxants are not actively reversed; the effects of action are terminated through the action of systemic pseudocholinesterase enzymes.

Non-depolarising muscle relaxants should not be reversed within 20 minutes of administration of the last dose. Neostigmine, 'Prostigmin' (Roche Products), is an effective antidote but because of muscarinic side effects, it should be given concurrently with atropine, even when further atropine has been used for premedication.

Neostigmine (2.5 mg) and atropine (1.2 mg) are mixed in a syringe. Small aliquots are given slowly, intravenously. After 1—2 minutes, ventilation is stopped for 10—15 seconds to see if spontaneous respiration will resume; if there is inadequate respiration, IPPV is resumed and the test repeated 1—2 minutes later. Further aliquots may be given every 3—5 minutes. The dose of neostigmine should be supra-maximal to ensure full reversal of all the effects of the relaxant; generally, doses of 0.1 mg/kg neostigmine should not be exceeded.

Great care should be taken to avoid hypoxia and hypercarbia whilst attempting to restore spontaneous respiration; ventilation should be supported whenever there is any doubt about the effectiveness of respiration.

SIGNS OF INCOMPLETE MUSCLE RELAXATION

1. Spontaneous respiratory movements in spite of IPPV.
2. Decreased chest compliance and increased resistance to ventilation.
3. Increased jaw muscle tone.

FAILURE TO RESTORE SPONTANEOUS RESPIRATION

Persistent apnoea may be caused by a number of factors;

1. Overdosage with relaxant.
   Repeated doses of suxamethonium produce a very resistant neuromuscular blockade.
2. Interference with excretion or elimination of relaxant.
   Liver and kidney disease can potentiate the duration of action of muscle relaxants.
3. Central depression due to overdose with premedicant and anaesthetic agents.
4. Electrolyte or acid-base imbalance.
5. Hypothermia.

Whilst apnoea persists, effective IPPV should be maintained. The use of analeptics and respiratory stimulants or excessive doses of neostigmine should be avoided. Intravenous fluid therapy should be instigated to encourage excretion of muscle relaxants and the patient should be kept warm.

FURTHER READING

HALL, L. W. (1982). Relaxant drugs in small animal anaesthesia. *Proc. Ass. Vet. An. G.Br. and Ir. Supplement to No. 10.* 144-155.

HALL, L. W. and CLARKE, K. W. (1991). *Veterinary Anaesthesia.* 9th edn. Balliere Tindall.

CHAPTER 10

ANAESTHESIA FOR CAESARIAN SECTION

B. M. Q. Weaver Ph.D., D.V.A., F.R.C.V.S.

OBJECTIVES

1. Safety and comfort of the mother.
2. Viable neonates.

SPECIAL REQUIREMENTS

1. An anaesthetic technique which will have a minimal adverse effect on the foetuses if live neonates are hoped for. Maintenance of optimal placental blood flow and blood oxygenation is important, as a reduction in placental blood flow is likely to mean reduced foetal oxygenation, which in turn leads to foetal bradycardia and acidosis.
2. A technique of anaesthesia which is suitable for the mother.
3. The state of health of the mother and foetuses in utero must be carefully assessed.

POSSIBLE ANAESTHETIC/ANALGESIC TECHNIQUES

a. Epidural analgesia.
b. Neuroleptanaesthesia.
c. General anaesthesia.

   a. **Epidural analgesia**

   Local analgesic solution is injected at the level of the lumbosacral vertebral junction. This technique has been used in the bitch, but the dose must be carefully noted.

   General disadvantages and dangers are:

   i. That some sedation may be required and, because the technique inevitably involves some depression of the sympathetic nervous system, there is a fall in blood pressure which may be detrimental to the oxygenation of the foetuses in utero, especially if haemorrhage occurs and fluid replacement therapy is not carried out.

   ii. That the local analgesic solution will be absorbed into the maternal systemic circulation and placental transfer will occur, the amount depending upon the degree of ionisation of the analgesic drug, the proportion of it which is protein bound and the rate at which it is metabolised. Bupivicaine is a preferable local anaesthetic to lignocaine for caesarian section because it is more highly ionised and is highly protein bound, so that the umbilical vein to maternal vein concentration ratio is quite low.

iii. That local analgesic drugs are weak bases and, if the condition of the foetuses deteriorates with the onset of metabolic acidosis, ions may become trapped in the foetal circulation and plasma binding will be reduced. These are factors conducive to increasing foetal toxicity.

iv. That the addition of adrenaline to the local analgesic solution reduces the dose required and prolongs the block, so that maternal blood levels and placental transfer are reduced. However, absorption of adrenaline into the maternal circulation can reduce placental blood flow.

v. That local analgesics increase myometrial toxicity thereby reducing placental perfusion.

b. **Neuroleptanaesthesia**

Neuroleptanaesthesia is a term used to describe narcosis brought about by the administration of a neuroleptic, ataractic or tranquilliser (e.g. acepromazine, fluanisone, droperidol) combined with one of the narcotic analgesic or opioid drugs, (e.g. morphine, pethidine, fentanyl, etorphine). Some commercially produced neuroleptanaesthetic mixtures are available; for example small animal Immobilon (etorphine with methotrimeprazine) and Hypnorm (fentanyl with fluanisone) (see Chapter 5).

Undesirable features of this method of anaesthesia include the following:

i. The drug combination reduces blood pressure in the bitch and causes severe respiratory depression. Thus, the foetuses are at risk of becoming hypoxic due to reduced placental blood flow and reduced oxygenation of the maternal blood. This can also be dangerous for the mother.

ii. Reversal of etorphine with diprenorphine 'Revivon' or fentanyl with naloxone 'Narcan neonatal' may not always be successful and the foetuses may succumb to depression due to incomplete reversal.

iii. Reversal of the narcotic analgesia in the bitch deprives her of any post operative analgesia and she, too, may succumb to depression if reversal subsequently proves to have been incomplete.

c. **General Anaesthesia**

Carefully managed general anaesthesia, which is balanced according to the individual's requirements, is the most satisfactory method.

Special considerations:

i. The condition of the mother needs to be carefully assessed and a detailed history of the case should be obtained.

ii. The operation may be elective or an emergency. If it is elective, the mother should be in a good state of health but if the procedure is an emergency, she may or may not be fit; indeed, she may be grossly weakened and dehydrated from a prolonged period of dystocia.

The physiological state of the mother will have changed during her pregnancy as follows:

1. The enlarging uterus will have pushed the diaphragm and heart forward.

2. The cardiac output will have increased and the systemic vascular resistance decreased.

3. The central venous pressure will have remained unaltered unless there has been pressure on the posterior vena cava.

4. Total blood volume will have increased but the haematocrit will have fallen and water and salt will have been retained to a greater extent than in the non-pregnant female.

5. Uterine perfusion will have increased dramatically.

6. Pulmonary blood volume will have increased.

7. Basal metabolic rate and oxygen consumption will have increased.

8. Pulmonary ventilation will have increased to meet the increased oxygen demands and, as a consequence, arterial carbon dioxide tension ($PaCO_2$) will have decreased from 40 mm Hg to about 35 mm Hg. It is important that it should not fall further during anaesthesia or foetal acidosis would result.

9. The Functional Residual Capacity (FRC) will have reduced, which means that alveolar gas concentrations can change more readily.

10. There will be hyperplasia of the anterior pituitary, thyroid and adrenocortical endocrine glands.

11. The minimal alveolar concentration (MAC) of inhalation anaesthetic agents will be reduced and resistance to injectable anaesthetic drugs will also be reduced.

iii. Placental transfer of almost any drug administered to the mother will occur. The extent of transfer will depend on:

1. lipid solubility
2. degree of ionisation
3. protein binding
4. molecular size
5. placental perfusion and placental drug metabolism

iv. Hypoxaemia must be avoided as this is detrimental to the mother and could be disastrous for the foetuses.

v. Vomiting or regurgitation may occur, especially if the operation is an emergency and the mother has recently eaten. If this does happen, there is a danger of acid stomach contents being inhaled and initiating Mendelson's syndrome (Mendelson 1946). There is also the risk of an oesophageal stricture developing. The airway must be protected with a cuffed endotracheal tube. Suction should be available and also an antacid solution of magnesium trisilicate or 0.3 M sodium citrate.

vi. Aorta-caval compression may occur. When the mother is placed in dorsal recumbency, the heavily gravid uterus may compress the abdominal aorta and vena cava. If this happens, maternal blood pressure will fall and placental blood flow will be reduced. The time that the mother is lying on her back before the abdomen is opened and the weight of the uterus is removed from these vessels, should be kept to a minimum.

vii. Haemorrhage from the uterus may persist if the organ does not involute satisfactorily after removal of the foetuses. This may be severe during deep halothane anaesthesia. As suturing of the uterus is being completed, oxytocin-S (0.2 – 1 ml) should be injected intramuscularly and the uterus should be seen to be involuting as it is replaced into the abdomen. Inspired concentrations of halothane should be kept to a minimum (i.e. not more than 0.5%).

ANAESTHETIC PROCEDURE

PREMEDICATION

Sedation, analgesia and the administration of an anticholinergic drug should be considered:-

Sedation and Analgesia

The need for this must be judged according to the condition and species of the mother:

- a. **The narcotic analgesics.**

    These cause neonatal respiratory depression, but pethidine does so less than most of the others and shifts the carbon dioxide respiratory response curve downwards much less than morphine. It is therefore, the agent of choice from this class of drug. Small doses may be given, (not more than 1 mg/kg) by subcutaneous injection about half an hour before anaesthesia is induced.

- b. **Acepromazine maleate.**

    A small dose may be given with the pethidine (not more than 0.03 mg/kg).

- c. Alternatively, **Diazepam** may be given, but in small doses (0.25—0.5 mg/kg) as it readily passes the placental barrier.

- d. **Medetomidine hydrochloride.**

    This agent is now licensed for use in the dog and cat. It is an α_2 adrenoceptor agonist inducing sedation and analgesia in a comparable manner to xylazine. Its use might be contemplated for caesarian section especially as the antagonist atipamezole hydrochloride is also available. However, the use of medetomidine for this purpose cannot be recommended since following injection of it, the heart rate falls rapidly and, as a consequence, it is to be expected that placental blood flow will be reduced with the concomitant risk of compromising foetal oxygenation.

Anticholinergic drugs

- a. **Atropine.**

    This does not cause sedation and may increase oxygen consumption. It may also increase foetal susceptibility to hypoxia. The normal response of the foetus to hypoxaemia is bradycardia, which slows down basal metabolic rate and reduces oxygen consumption. If atropine is given, this bradycardia is reversed and the safety feature is lost. Atropine also relaxes the lower oesophageal sphincter of the mother, facilitating possible gastro-oesophageal reflux, which could lead to a post anaesthetic oesophageal stricture.

    However, atropine reverses bradycardia in the mother, which is very serious. Thus, it should not be given as a routine, but always be ready to give if necessary (0.02 mg/kg I/V, repeated if bradycardia is not reversed).

- b. **Glycopyrronium,** 'Robinul' (Robins).

    This is an alternative anticholinergic agent (0.01 mg/kg) and is preferable if such an agent is required. It passes the blood-brain and placental barriers only poorly, is long acting (several hours) and can raise the gastric pH.

INDUCTION

If the mother is weak or very placid, she may accept a gently applied mask. Anaesthesia can then be induced by inhalation using; nitrous oxide and oxygen (minimum 30%) with halothane up to 2%. If, however, the mother is alert, the induction should be carried out by intravenous injection of a rapidly acting anaesthetic which has a short duration of action. The following agents can be considered:

- a. Thiopentone sodium 'Intraval'
- b. Methohexitone 'Brietal'
- c. Alphaxalone and alphadolone 'Saffan'
- d. Propofol 'Rapinovet'
- e. Ketamine hydrochloride 'Vetalar'

a / b. **Thiopentone and Methohexitone** act rapidly, i.e. they pass the blood-brain barrier quickly, but this means that they also pass the placental barrier just as readily. However, only the non-ionised molecule can readily pass biological membranes and, at normal blood pH, only about half the barbiturate exists in this form. They have a short duration of action due to a redistribution from the brain to other parts of the body rather than to rapid metabolism. They are therefore suitable for induction of anaesthesia for caesarian section **provided** only a sleep inducing single injection is given. Methohexitone is preferable to thiopentone as it has a shorter duration of action.

'Saffan' and 'Rapinovet' act as rapidly as the barbiturates and have the advantage of being rapidly metabolised.

c. **Alphaxalone and alphadolone** 'Saffan' can be used in the cat but may initiate hypersensitivity reactions. It should **not** be used in the **dog** because, in this species, undesirable reactions are especially liable to occur.

d. **Propofol** 'Rapinovet' is a recently introduced, rapidly metabolised intravenous anaesthetic and is therefore the induction agent of choice, but it is likely to pass the placental barrier readily and so should be only used for induction.

e. **Ketamine** 'Vetalar' can be used to induce anaesthesia in the cat but is **not** suitable for the **dog**. Only a small dose (not more than 5 mg/kg) should be given, intravenously if possible. Ketamine raises the maternal blood pressure but does not reduce placental blood flow and it is analgesic.

MAINTENANCE

As soon as the mother is asleep, her airway must be protected with a cuffed endotracheal tube and anaesthesia maintained by controlled inhalation. At the present time, halothane with oxygen is the most likely agent to be used, but the inspired concentration must be kept minimal (i.e. not more than 0.5% if possible). Isoflurane, having a lower tissue solubility and being less depressant to the circulation, could be preferable to halothane but, at present, it is much more expensive. Nitrous oxide can be added to the gas mixture and its analgesic properties reduce the halothane or isoflurane requirement. Care must be taken to see that the inspired oxygen does not fall below 50%.

POSITIONING THE MOTHER FOR SURGERY

The mother must be moved carefully and gently turned into the supine position for midline laparotomy. The weight of the gravid uterus may compress the posterior vena cava and possibly also the aorta and either factor can compromise placental blood flow. Thus **before** turning the mother, a vein should be cannulated and a slow intravenous infusion of a balanced electrolyte solution commenced. In addition, the pulse, heart rate and, if possible, the blood pressure should be monitored.

MUSCLE RELAXANT DRUGS

These drugs may be used as adjuncts to anaesthesia, especially if it is thought desirable or it becomes necessary to control pulmonary ventilation by intermittent positive pressure (IPPV). The non-depolarising muscle relaxants are highly ionised at physiological pH and are poorly lipid soluble so that placental transfer is limited. Nevertheless, it does occur and so only minimal doses should be given. Atracurium besylate 'Tracrium' is relatively short acting and is the relaxant of choice at present. If ventilation is controlled by IPPV, care must be taken as indicated earlier, not to hyperventilate and reduce the arterial carbon dioxide of the mother (already lowered during pregnancy) as this would lead to foetal acidosis due to direct vasoconstriction of the uterine vessels and maternal cardiac output might be reduced which would lead to foetal hypoxia.

Care must also be taken to ensure that the mother is unconscious for the whole duration of action of the muscle relaxant drug.

MONITORING

Monitoring the physiological status of the mother during the operation is important, for the safety of both mother and foetuses. Monitoring equipment is continually improving and much can be done at the present time non-invasively.

For example:

> Feeling the pulse and hearing the heart beating via an oesophageal stethoscope.
>
> An electrocardiograph can continuously display the electrical activity of the heart.
>
> Measurement of the blood pressure by oscillimetry can now be carried out non-invasively with equipment, such as the 'Dinamap' (Critikon), and an intermittent display of the systolic, diastolic and mean blood pressures and the heart rate, can be obtained.
>
> An oxygen monitor, such as the 'Oxycheck' (Critikon), can be used to check the mother's inspired oxygen concentration.
>
> A rapid response carbon dioxide analyser, such as the 'Normocap' (Datex), can check on the level of expired carbon dioxide.
>
> A volatile anaesthetic analyser, such as the 'Normac' (Datex), can be used to monitor the inspired concentration of halothane or isoflurane.

NEONATAL RESUSCITATION

1. A warm, dry container with suitable bedding should be ready to receive the newborn animals.

2. It is most urgent, after birth, for the lungs to expand and for a full cardiac output to be sent to them.

3. The first breath requires unusual effort as the foetal lung contains fluid and the first breath has to overcome surface tension at fluid-air interspaces and a high transpulmonary pressure is generated, albeit briefly. After the first breath, a functional residual capacity must be built up to prevent collapse.

4. To assist the neonate to take its first breath, the nostrils, mouth and pharynx should be gently cleared of fluid. It should be placed in a slightly head down position to assist drainage and the ribs and nostrils gently stimulated with a warm towel.

5. The neonate's condition should be assessed according to the following signs:-

    Presence of reflex response to stimulation

    Palpable heart beat

    Respiratory effort

    Muscle tone

    Colour of mucous membranes

6. If the neonates are weak, they should be given oxygen enriched air to breathe.

7. The neonates should be united with their mother as soon as she is able to care for them.

SUMMARY

Caesarian section in small animals is preferably carried out under general anaesthesia. Provided this is carefully managed, the operation can be carried out with minimal discomfort to the mother and any viable foetuses she has, can be expected to survive. It is important to bear in mind the factors mentioned earlier, which influence placental transfer of drugs and, in addition, factors which contribute to neonatal depression.

For example:

a. A high concentration of drugs in the maternal circulation leading to a high concentration of drugs in the foetal circulation.

b. Respiratory depression.

c. A fall in maternal blood pressure.

d. A reduction in placental blood flow.

FURTHER READING

MENDELSON, C. L. (1946). The aspiration of stomach contents into the lungs during obstetric anaesthesia. *The American Journal of Obstetrics and Gynaecology.* Vol 52, 191.

DODMAN, N. H. (1979). Anaesthesia for caesarian section in the dog and cat; a review. *J. small Anim. Pract.* **20**, 449.

JOSHUA, J. O. (1956). Epidural anaesthesia for caesarian section. *Vet. Rec.* **68**, 801.

REILLY, J. (1983). Anaesthesia for caesarian section in small animals and the mare. *Anaesthesia & Intensive Care, University of Sydney Refresher Course for the Veterinarian, Proceeding No. 62.* 131.

CHAPTER 11
ANAESTHESIA FOR THORACIC SURGERY

G. J. Brouwer B.Vet.Med., B.Sc., D.V.A., M.R.C.V.S.

Thoracotomy may be necessary for a number of reasons including exploratory investigations, retrieval of oesophageal foreign bodies, correction of vascular anomalies (e.g. patent ductus arteriosus), lobectomy and cardiac surgery. Many of the principles of thoracic anaesthesia apply equally to repair of diaphragmatic rupture although, conventionally, these are repaired through laparotomy incision.

PRE-OPERATIVE EVALUATION AND PREPARATION

Before any thoracic procedure, the patient should be thoroughly examined and evaluated. Care should be taken during the clinical examination (which may include radiography), that the patient does not become distressed, since cardio-pulmonary function is likely to be compromised; a source of oxygen should be readily available.

In order to keep anaesthetic and surgical time to an absolute minimum, preclipping of the surgical site is to be recommended, provided that this is tolerated by the patient. Further, the preplacement of both a jugular and a peripheral (cephalic) vein catheter is advisable. The jugular catheter is used to administer fluids before, during and after anaesthesia, whilst the smaller catheter is used to administer drugs intravenously.

PREMEDICATION

Most routinely used premedicant drugs have been used for thoracic anaesthesia. The choice will be dictated by the clinical condition of the patient, the nature of any cardio-pulmonary compromise and the known side effects of the preferred drugs. The judicious use of atropine, acetylpromazine and pethidine, would meet most requirements. Once premedicated, the patient should be continuously observed (see Chapter 5).

INDUCTION

Induction of anaesthesia for thoracic surgery is perhaps the time of greatest danger; physiological compensatory mechanisms are suddenly altered by the onset of anaesthesia endangering the supply of blood and oxygen to vital areas. Pre-oxygenation of the patient, if it is tolerated without causing distress, is to be recommended.

Induction of anaesthesia by volatile agent given by face mask is too slow and readily leads to induction excitement, hypoxia and hypercarbia; it cannot be recommended. An intravenous induction using thiopentone or propofol is generally safe; doses should be kept low and endotracheal intubation performed as soon as possible. The patient should then be quickly connected to an anaesthetic circuit delivering oxygen only; if spontaneous respiration is inadequate, the patient should be briefly ventilated to ensure adequate oxygenation.

MAINTENANCE

During surgery, the chest will be open to the atmosphere and therefore the way in which anaesthesia is maintained will be determined by:-

1. the need to sustain unconsciousness and unresponsiveness to surgery and
2. the need to provide intermittent positive pressure ventilation (IPPV) to supply oxygen to and remove carbon dioxide from the lungs.

Two main approaches to maintaining anaesthesia for thoracic procedures can be adopted.

Firstly, IPPV can be used to provide oxygen only whilst anaesthesia is maintained by incremental doses of intravenous anaesthetic. This is a very safe approach; good oxygenation can be assured, but recovery from anaesthesia can become delayed if incremental doses of intravenous anaesthetic have a cumulative effect (e.g. thiopentone). The level of anaesthesia can be less rapidly altered in response to the requirements of surgery.

Secondly, IPPV can be used to provide both oxygenation and anaesthesia by way of concurrent use of oxygen and volatile anaesthetics (e.g. nitrous oxide and halothane). The use of volatile anaesthetics allows anaesthesia to be more finely regulated and, since cummulative effects are less, recovery from anaesthesia can be more rapid. Force ventilating with volatile anaesthetic agents can be very dangerous and only very low concentrations are usually necessary. Further, the technique also demands a thorough understanding of how the ventilating equipment actually functions since this influences what concentrations of anaesthetic gas are likely to be delivered to the patient.

Whenever IPPV is to be practised, endotracheal intubation of the patient is essential. Ventilation by mask is technically difficult to sustain and invariably is associated with simultaneous inflation of the stomach.

Typical techniques.

There are many ways in which anaesthesia can be successfully maintained during thoracic surgery, depending upon the range of drugs and equipment available and the experience of the anaesthetist. Some commonly used protocols may include the following:-

CAT
1. Induction with propofol, followed by maintenance using incremental doses of propofol. IPPV using oxygen administered via a paediatric to-and-fro system
2. Induction with thiopentone. IPPV and maintenance with 2L/min oxygen plus 2L/min nitrous oxide and 0.3% halothane delivered via a modified Ayre's T-piece.

DOG
1. Induction with thiopentone; maintenance with incremental doses of thiopentone or methohexitone. IPPV with oxygen delivered via a to-and-fro system.
2. Induction with thiopentone. IPPV and maintenance using 0.8% halothane in oxygen delivered via a circle system. The spill-off valve should be partially open and a continuous flow (1L/min) of oxygen/halothane should be administered to the circuit.
3. Induction with thiopentone. IPPV and maintenance using 50% oxygen plus 50% nitrous oxide plus 0.3% halothane using an appropriate non-rebreathing system (e.g. Mini-Vent, Manley Ventilator or Flomasta Ventilator). For a 25kg dog, a fresh gas flow rate of 6–9 L/min would be needed.

The Stephens anaesthetic machine has an in-circuit vaporiser. With the vaporiser on, IPPV tends to cause a very rapid build-up of volatile agent within the circuit. Its use during IPPV requires very great care and it is probably better if the vaporiser is emptied and the circle system simply used to deliver oxygen alone in these circumstances.

Ventilating Pattern

Patients undergoing thoracic surgery will often have pre-existing ventilation-perfusion problems which will be compounded by anaesthesia. Once the chest is open, there will be a tendency for lungs to collapse, which will be encouraged by surgical packs placed inside the thorax. Therefore, there will be a trend in these patients to develop hypoxia and hypercarbia; for this reason HYPERVENTILATION rather than hypoventilation, should be the aim.

The ventilatory rate should mimick that of the normal animal at rest; dogs, 12—20 breaths/minute; cats, 20—30 breaths/minute. The tidal volume should be sufficient to produce good chest movement with the chest closed and satisfactory lung expansion with the chest open; tidal volumes of 15—20 mls/kg are usually suggested. The ventilatory pressure should be the lowest practicable to avoid alveolar damage and restriction of venous return to the heart and yet achieve adequate lung inflation; pressures of 10—25 cm of water (GENTLE HAND PRESSURE) are commonly used. The inspiratory to expiratory time ratio should be about 1:2; a rapid inflation and a longer expiratory pause appears to provide an optimal pattern.

Muscle relaxants.

The use of neuromuscular blocking drugs (muscle relaxants) for administering IPPV is not mandatory, although it is to be recommended, particularly in the dog. The use of muscle relaxants achieves good surgical conditions at lighter levels of anaesthesia and the reduced amounts of anaesthetic lead to less side effects in patients that are at greater risk. Further, muscle relaxants reduce resistance to mechanical ventilation and, therefore, lower inflation pressures can be used during IPPV. The use of muscle relaxants is further discussed in Chapter 9.

Monitoring.

The monitoring of anaesthesia during thoracic surgery should be particularly vigilant. The safety of the patient is as much in the hands of the surgeon, since rough handling of the lungs, the heart, the major vascular vessels and the numerous thoracic nerves, can have profound effects upon the circulation and upon ventilation. Should sudden changes occur, particularly to the circulation, surgery should be temporarily suspended whilst stability is re-established. Increased resistance to ventilation can often be attributed to over-zealous packing-off of lungs or inadvertent lung torsions; these should be corrected at once.

The anaesthetist should also be aware of the surgeon's needs; the ventilatory pattern may need to be adjusted or even temporarily suspended during periods of delicate surgery so as to prevent tissue movement or damage by instruments.

The rate and quality of the pulse will be particularly important as will be the colour of the mucous membranes to ensure that circulation and ventilation remain adequate throughout surgery and anaesthesia.

Fluid Therapy.

Fluid losses during thoracic surgery can be considerable. There is increased fluid loss during IPPV through use of dry anaesthetic gases, and there is marked evaporative loss from within the thorax whilst it is open to the atmosphere. These losses are compounded by blood losses incurred during surgery. For maintenance, fluids need to be administered typically at the rate of 10 mls/kg/hour; a greater rate will be needed if pulse quality deteriorates or if haemorrhage becomes significant. Half the fluid volume should be given as a colloid (plasma substitute) and the other half as crystalloid (dextrose-saline or hartmanns solution).

Fluid therapy will need to be carefully monitored where there is pre-existing cardiac failure or where there is a suspected increase in right-heart pressure (e.g. pulmonary artery stenosis). In such cases, monitoring of arterial and central venous pressure may be specifically indicated.

Hypothermia.

Prolonged surgery and anaesthesia, exposure of the thoracic organs to the atmosphere and ventilating with cold anaesthetic gases, contribute towards significant heat loss. Hypothermia during thoracic surgery is commonly encountered and it is important to reduce this problem as much as possible. Adequate planning can keep anaesthesia time to the minimum; the operating theatre should be warm and the patient placed on a heated pad or water-bed; operating drapes should be kept as dry as possible and intravenous fluids should be warmed before administration. Post-operatively, the patient should be placed in a warm area, kept scrupulously dry and given warm intravenous fluid. Gentle heat provided by a hair dryer can be used to restore body heat more rapidly. Hypothermia is the commonest cause of delayed recovery from anaesthesia.

CHEST DRAINAGE

The air trapped within the thorax when the chest wall is closed needs to be removed since pneumothorax will compromise ventilation regardless of whether IPPV is being applied or whether respiration is spontaneous. Over inflation of the lungs as the last suture is being placed to seal the chest, rarely expels all the air and risks damage to alveoli; reinflation of collapsed lung tissue is also difficult this way without causing lung damage. Aspiration of the trapped air using a needle or catheter passed through the chest wall risks traumatising the lungs and, if repeated, could introduce infection.

The preferred method, even in a cat, is to place a chest drain under direct vision before closure of the thorax. The drain should be a purpose made catheter of an appropriate size, be sterile and cause minimal tissue reaction. It is commonly placed in the lower third of the chest with a sufficient length within the chest to prevent its tip from coming out of the thoracic cavity. It is passed subcutaneously over at least two rib spaces before entering the thorax at a site away from the thoracotomy incision. For additional safety, the drain is anchored to the skin.

Once the chest wall is closed, the air within the thorax is **gently** aspirated using a syringe and three way tap or using a water-seal bottle attached to a low pressure suction machine. Suction is continued until slight resistance is first encountered.

The principal period of aspiration will be at the conclusion of surgery, but suction may need to be repeated 1–3 hourly during recovery and subsequently at 8 hourly intervals until no further air is removed or the patient is able to ventilate adequately. The chest drain is commonly removed within 8 hours of recovery from anaesthesia and it is rarely necessary to retain a drain beyond 48 hours. The chest drain should never be left unattended in the conscious animal. Where continual supervision is not possible, the drain should be plugged and bandaged in place against the chest wall so that the patient cannot damage or remove it.

RECOVERY AND POST-OPERATIVE CARE

Towards the end of surgery, anaesthesia should be lightened as much as possible and spontaneous respiration re-established. IPPV should be periodically stopped whilst the patient's own respiratory effort is assessed. Failure to resume respiration may be due to the residual effect of muscle relaxants, the residual action of anaesthetic drugs or hypothermia. Apnoea should not be tolerated for more than a few seconds and IPPV **must** be continued until the patient is able to support his own respiration; an inability to maintain good oxygenation in the face of high inspired oxygen concentrations suggests a persisting pneumothorax.

Thoracic surgery is associated with considerable post-operative pain. Potent analgesics are required and these should be administered just prior to resumption of consciousness. Given at this stage, lower doses can be used to achieve good analgesia during the post-operative period. Morphine, pethidine and buprenorphine are the drugs of choice, and if used at clinical doses, respiratory depression is unlikely to be a significant problem (see Chapter 4).

Post-operative radiography is often of value after thoracic surgery. The extent of any residual pneumothorax can be assessed and the location of the thoracic drain confirmed. Further radiographs are indicated if the condition of the patient deteriorates unexpectedly.

During recovery, the patient should be monitored intensively. The routine parameters, such as body temperature, pulse rate and quality, capillary refill time, mucous membrane colour and respiratory rate, should be initially assessed and recorded every 15 minutes. As the patient stabilises, the monitoring intervals can be extended. Fluid therapy should be continued to establish a good urinary output. Chest drainage will be repeated periodically; the volume of air or the nature of any fluid aspirated, can be noted. Only when the animal is fully conscious, able to sit up and preferably able to walk about, may it be left reasonably unsupervised.

FURTHER READING

CLARKE, K. W. (1977). Anaesthesia for open chest surgery. *J small Anim Pract.* **18** 585-590.
HALL, L. W. and CLARKE, K. W. (1991). *Veterinary Anaesthesia.* 9th edn. Balliere Tindall.

CHAPTER 12

ANAESTHESIA FOR OPHTHALMIC SURGERY

B. M. Q. Weaver Ph.D., D.V.A., F.R.C.V.S.

REQUIREMENTS

1. A quiet stress free induction of anaesthesia.

2. No movement during the operation to minimise any risk of damage to the eye during delicate precision surgery.

3. A quiet emergence from anaesthesia to minimise trauma to the eye. This is especially important.

4. For intra-ocular surgery, a low intra-ocular pressure is required. Thus, drugs known to raise the intra-ocular pressure should not be used (e.g. ketamine and the muscle relaxant suxamethonium). Every attempt should be made to prevent the occurrence of vomiting or coughing and hypertension should be avoided.

Factors to be considered:

a. The age, metabolic status (presence of any concurrent disease, e.g. diabetes mellitus) and temperament of the patient.

b. The operation to be performed may be elective, for example, lens extraction for cataract or an entropion in which case the patient can be prepared for surgery; its general condition can be assessed and treated if necessary, and food can be withheld for 6–12 hours to allow the stomach to empty. It may, however, be an emergency, for example, extraction of a luxated lens with glaucoma developing, removal of a foreign body or repair of an injury. In these cases food may have been recently ingested and special care must be taken to protect the airway. A cuffed endotracheal tube should be used and suction should be available in case there is a regurgitation of stomach contents. In addition, the animal's condition must be assessed as anaesthesia proceeds.

c. Any drug therapy currently in use to treat the ophthalmic condition or to be used during the operation, should be considered. This is because agents are absorbed into the systemic circulation if instilled into the conjuctival sac, or they may have been administered systemically.

They may include:

i. Atropine. This parasympathetic depressant drug may be given to induce mydriasis. It should not be given routinely as part of the anaesthetic protocol but either atropine or preferably glycopyrronium, should be ready to be given, if necessary, e.g. to counteract bradycardia, which may be due to vagal stimulation occurring via the oculo-cardiac reflex initiated as a result of pressure on the eyeball or traction on the extra-ocular muscles of the orbit.

ii. Drugs used in the treatment of glaucoma:

1. Sympathomimetics such as adrenaline or phenylephrine, which reduce the production of aqueous humor. These agents may initiate cardiac arrhythmias in the presence of halothane.

2. Miotics may be used to facilitate aqueous drainage. For example, the cholinergic agent pilocarpine and anticholinesterases such as ecothiopate ('Phospholine Iodide') or physostigmine (eserine).

N.B. Drug acting on the pupil, e.g. atropine, miotics and sympathomimetics prevent the use of pupillary size in assessing anaesthetic depth.

Drugs which decrease plasma cholinesterase mean that a serious prolongation of the ester-type local anaesthetics, such as procaine or of suxamethonium, could occur.

3. Diuretics

a. Carbonic anhydrase inhibitors such as dichlorphenamide ('Daranide') and acetazolamide ('Diamox'). These drugs suppress aqueous humor formation and they are given systemically, as they are ineffective applied locally. Their use may lead to considerable electrolyte loss, in particular potassium, via the kidneys.

b. Osmotic diuretics such as mannitol or 50% sucrose.

When diuretics have been given to reduce intra-ocular pressure, a slow intravenous infusion of a balanced electrolyte solution should be administered peri-operatively to compensate for the fluid and electrolyte loss.

4. Beta-blocking drugs are used in human patients to reduce intra-ocular pressure. They do so without constricting the pupil. They are not often used in animals at present, but if they were to be, systemic effects, such as bronchoconstriction, could occur.

iii. Corticosteroid agents are often used in treating ocular conditions. If they are being used, then the therapy should be sustained during anaesthesia, since the animal's ability to release its own corticosteroids in response to stress, may be reduced.

ANALGESIC OR ANAESTHETIC PROCEDURES

Topical Analgesia

The application of a local analgesic agent on to the cornea or into the conjunctival sac will desensitise the cornea and conjunctiva. This may facilitate the examination of a painful eye, assist in the removal of a foreign body or allow a very minor operation to be performed. The most commonly used agents are the eye drop preparations of lignocaine (4%), oxybuprocaine (0.4%) or proxymetacaine (0.5%). These agents are short acting, their effects wearing off within half an hour. Eye drops of amethocaine (0.5–1%) will bring about a more prolonged desensitisation.

Local Infiltration

This might be considered for minor surgery, e.g. removal of a small tumour. A small amount of 1% or 2% lignocaine being injected where an incision is to be made.

REGIONAL NERVE BLOCKS

Supra-orbital block

The supra-orbital nerve supplies sensation to the upper eyelid and so it could be blocked using 1% or 2% lignocaine for minor surgery in that region.

Auriculo-palpebral block

The auriculo-palpebral nerve is a branch of the facial motor nerve and supplies the muscles of the eyelid. Blocking it does not produce any desensitisation and thus is only likely to be considered to prevent the animal closing its lids tightly and applying pressure to the orbit, e.g. after surgery or to assist in the removal of a foreign body (see Chapter 8).

Retrobulbar block

This is brought about by depositing local analgesic solution, e.g. 1% lignocaine, behind the orbit. It is only likely to be of use during general anaesthesia where surgery on the eye is impossible because of retraction of the orbit. The approach is via the conjunctival sac using a small (25g) needle to minimise the risk of haemorrhage and damage to the optic and other nerves traversing the retrobulbar space. Care must be taken not to inject the solution into a blood vessel and the amount of lignocaine injected must be noted to avoid the possibility of toxicity as it is absorbed into the circulation. This block reduces intra-ocular pressure and causes mydriasis.

GENERAL ANAESTHESIA.

A carefully balanced general anaesthetic should be administered having as its aim a quiet induction, maintenance of a steady state of anaesthesia with a low intra-ocular pressure and a quiet emergence to consciousness.

Premedication

Sedation with acepromazine (0.05 mg/kg) is usually satisfactory, preferably mixed with a narcotic analgesic e.g. pethidine (1 mg/kg).

Induction

Induction is by a slow intravenous injection of a rapidly acting agent having a short duration of action:

> **Thiopentone** (1.25–2.5%) is quite suitable but doses should be kept minimal (<10 mg/kg) otherwise recovery may be associated with incoordination and risk of trauma to the eye which has been operated on.
>
> **Methohexitone** ('Brietal'). Quite suitable at a dose of not more than 5 mg/kg.
>
> **Propofol** ('Rapinovet'). Very suitable. A dose of about 4 mg/kg will induce anaesthesia after pre-anaesthetic sedation, but more can be given if necessary. This agent is rapidly metabolised and not redistributed like the barbiturates, so that recovery will not be associated with a prolonged period of incoordination. It should be given cautiously and the heart rate checked for possible bradycardia.

MAINTENANCE

Once anaesthesia is induced, the trachea must be intubated with a suitable cuffed endotracheal tube without stimulating coughing or retching and with minimal vagal or sympathetic stimulation. This can be achieved fairly easily in dogs, especially if use is made of a topical application of 2% lignocaine. If anaesthesia is not deep enough after induction, inhalation of halothane in oxygen and nitrous oxide via a mask, can be carried out until the animal is relaxed. In the cat, endotracheal intubation after a barbiturate is liable to initiate undesirable reflex responses, but inhalation of halothane in oxygen with nitrous oxide via a mask as with the dog, will facilitate the procedure. Alternatively, a non-depolarising muscle relaxant such as atracurium ('Tracrium'), could be given after induction and pre-oxygenation, ventilation then being controlled by intermittent positive pressure (IPPV).

Anaesthesia should be maintained by controlled inhalation administered via a suitable breathing system.

Halothane, enflurane, isoflurane or methoxyflurane, may be used as each of these agents reduces intra-ocular pressure. In the human, isoflurane has been shown to be preferable to halothane for cataract surgery (Inglis, 1988). Nitrous oxide is a useful adjunct to the use of any of these agents provided the inspired oxygen concentration does not fall below 30%. It should be discontinued, however, if it is necessary to inject air into the eye, to replace intra-orbital content.

Ventilation may be spontaneous, in which case care must be taken to see that respiration is not depressed, or it may be controlled by the anaesthetist with the aid of a non-depolarising muscle relaxant, in which case slight hyperventilation is an advantage.

Muscle Relaxant Drugs

Depolarising muscle relaxants should not be used as these will initially cause contraction of the retrobulbar muscles increasing intraocular pressure and retraction of the eyeball.

Non-depolarising muscle relaxants such as atracurium, mentioned above, can be used as part of the anaesthetic technique. With such a procedure, the eyeball does not rotate and the cornea remains central facilitating corneal and intraocular surgery but the technique requires ensuring that the required level of anaesthesia is maintained and respiration must be controlled by IPPV. Furthermore any residual curarisation at the end of the operation must be reversed with atropine and neostigmine.

Monitoring

Monitoring end-tidal carbon dioxide concentration enables the efficiency of pulmonary ventilation to be checked.

Monitoring the blood pressure using a non-invasive oscillometric method, e.g. 'Dinamap' (Critikon), is useful as this can influence the intra-ocular pressure. It should not be allowed to rise during surgery and can usually be controlled by varying the inspired concentration of the volatile anaesthetic.

If diuretics have been used, serum potassium should be monitored. If the patient is diabetic, hourly monitoring of the blood sugar should be carried out.

FURTHER READING

CRISPIN, S. M. (1981) Anaesthesia for ophthalmic surgery. *Proc. Ass. Vet. An. G. Br. & Ir.* **9**, 171.

INGLIS, M. S. (1988). Halothane and Isoflurane — a comparison for cataract surgery. *Today's Anaesthetist,* **3**, No. 1, 10.

BEDFORD, P. G. C. (1988). Condition of the eyelids in the dog. *J. small. Anim. Pract.* **29**, No. 7, 417-418.

SANSOM, J. (1988). Antibacterials in the treatment of ocular infections. *J. small Anim. Pract.* **29**, No. 7, 487-492.

CLUTTON, R. E. BOYD, C., RICHARDS, D. L. S. and SCHWINK, K. (1988). Significance of the oculocardiac reflex during ophthalmic surgery in the dog. *J. small Anim. Pract.* **29**, No. 9, 573.

CHAPTER 13
ANAESTHESIA OF GERIATRICS AND NEONATES

A. E. Waterman B.V.Sc., Ph.D., D.V.A., M.R.C.V.S.

ANAESTHESIA OF THE GERIATRIC DOG OR CAT

The definition of what constitutes a geriatric animal is very difficult since animals, like people, vary enormously in the rate at which their fitness and agility decline. However, for the most part, one would start to consider that dogs over 10 years of age, and cats over 12 years, need special consideration.

PATHOPHYSIOLOGICAL CONSIDERATIONS

1. Geriatric animals have reduced ability to metabolise and excrete drugs and, while renal function is usually normal, renal reserves are commonly decreased so that any episode of hypotension or hypovolaemia can have disastrous consequences.
2. Plasma protein binding of drugs can alter with age, as do the pharmacokinetics of many drugs, so that their volumes of distribution and clearance rates decrease.
3. Aged animals frequently suffer from some degree of heart disease. Even if they are not in congestive heart failure, the presence of incompetent heart valves will reduce cardiac reserves so that it is likely that both cardiac output will be reduced and the circulation time will be prolonged.

PRE-OPERATIVE MANAGEMENT

Careful consideration should be given to these patients. The heart and lungs should be auscultated and the owner questioned carefully as to the animal's exercise tolerance.

The possibility that the animal's renal functional reserves may be reduced, should be considered. If possible blood urea and creatinine levels should be checked pre-operatively and fluid intake should NOT be restricted.

Choice of technique

Whatever the technique chosen, there are a few guidelines which should be followed:

1. Periods of hypovolaemia, hypotension or hypoxia should be avoided.
2. A balanced regime rather than a single drug should be chosen so as to reduce dosages and minimise side effects.
3. Drugs that require extensive metabolism for cessation of their action should be avoided.
4. If possible, drugs, the effects of which may be reversed by a specific antagonist if necessary, should be used.

TECHNIQUE

Premedication.

The use of high doses of phenothiazines should be avoided. However, judicious use of the drug acepromazine in low doses (0.03 – 0.05 mg/kg), alone or in combination with an analgesic, can be most useful. Acepromazine has a protective effect against dysrhythmias and will also calm the animal, but the hypotensive effect of this drug must be a borne in mind during anaesthesia when fluids may need to be given intravenously. Pethidine is the analgesic choice for elderly animals, by virtue of its short duration of action and lack of unpleasant side effects. A dose of 1mg/kg for premedication in combination with Acepromazine, or 2 mg/kg when given alone, should be used.

Anticholinergic drugs should not be administered as a matter of routine in these animals, since tachycardia imposes a considerable extra work burden on the myocardium. If there is a likelihood of vagal stimulation or excessive salivation glycopyrrolate should be used in preference to atropine (see chapter 5).

Induction

1. A short acting intravenous agent such as thiopentone, methohexitone, propofol (or 'Saffan' in cats), should be chosen. Pentobarbitone, which is long lasting and needs to be metabolised, should be avoided. Since circulation time is often slow, the drug should be given more slowly than usual and reduced dosage requirements should be anticipated.

2. In ill, old animals, it may be preferable to use halothane or isoflurane administered in a N_2O/O_2 gas mixture via a mask alone or following a 'sleep' dose of thiopentone or propofol. This is often possible if the animal is first premedicated with a combination of acepromazine and pethidine.

Maintenance

1. Hypoxia should be guarded against, and therefore, an inspired concentration of at least 30 – 40% of oxygen should always be used.

2. Hypotension should be avoided by keeping the anaesthesia as light as possible and by setting up an I/V infusion to give fluids as necessary.

3. The use of an anaesthetic regime employing a muscle relaxant, intermittent positive pressure ventilation (IPPV) and an infusion of an analgesic such as fentanyl, combined with very low inspired concentrations of halothane or isoflurane in N_2O/O_2, has much to recommend it. However, most old animals will tolerate a regime of spontaneous respiration and a volatile agent, as long as hypoventilation is avoided.

4. The choice of volatile agent is usually dictated by availability and expense. Isoflurane would be the preferred agent, but is expensive. Halothane, although it causes hypotension and predisposes to arrhythmias, is widely used and is safe. Methoxyflurane can also be used but recovery from this agent is slow and some of its metabolites are potentially nephrotoxic, although no fully documented cases of renal failure have been recorded in dogs.

5. Body temperature should be monitored and hypothermia avoided. This is especially vital in old cats.

6. In patients with heart disease caution should be exercised in administering excess sodium. Therefore, 'normal' (0.9%) saline solution should be avoided. Balanced polyionic solutions should be used instead and losses replaced on a volume for volume basis.

7. Pulse, respiration, colour of mucous membranes and anaesthetic depth should be monitored closely.

Recovery

1. Body temperature should be monitored and steps taken to remedy hypothermia.

2. Respiration, pulse rate and volume should be monitored and a close check kept on the colour of the mucous membranes.

3. An I/V line should be kept open for drug or fluid administration.

4. Additional oxygen should be available and given if needed.

5. Antagonists should be administered if necessary.

6. Analgesia should be provided; pethidine at 2 – 3 mg/kg I/M, will provide 2 – 3 hours analgesia.

FURTHER READING

EVANS, A.T. (1981) Anaesthesia for the geriatric patient. *Vet. Clinics North America,*
Vol II, 653-667.

ANAESTHESIA OF THE PAEDIATRIC DOG AND CAT

The first twelve weeks of life may be regarded as the paediatric period. Neonatal puppies and kittens (the neonatal period is 0 – 2 weeks), are extremely immature but rarely require anaesthesia. However, from four weeks onwards, infant pups or kittens may well need to be anaesthetised for a variety of reasons.

PATHOPHYSIOLOGICAL CONSIDERATIONS

1. Paediatric patients have a large surface area to body weight ratio and a high basal metabolic rate (B.M.R.). In addition, they lack subcutaneous fat, have a higher obligatory heat loss, a relative inability to produce heat by shivering or non-shivering thermogenesis and have a poorly developed thermoregulatory mechanism. They are, therefore, very susceptible to hypothermia under anaesthesia as heat losses increase and production decreases.

2. Young animals have an immature hepatic microsomal enzyme system so that detoxification of drugs is limited.

3. Renal function is not fully developed in paediatric animals so that they are neither able to produce very concentrated nor dilute urine in response to water deprivation or fluid overload, nor excrete acid urine.

4. Paediatric animals also have a higher percentage body water than adults and the ratio of extra cellular fluid (E.C.F.) to intra cellular fluid (I.C.F.), is greater. They have a high rate of water turnover which makes them prime candidates for dehydration. Fluid balance must, therefore, be monitored closely.

5. Pulmonary function is not fully developed in neonates. They have fewer alveoli and less surfactant in their lungs than adults. Thus, there is a reduced area of lung available for gas exchange and so they tend to compensate by breathing at a faster rate and a higher minute volume. Normal regulatory responses to hypoxia and hypercarbia are also poorly developed, yet, because of their high B.M.R., they have a high O_2 requirement (twice that of adults).

6. The high affinity of foetal haemoglobin for oxygen, reduces the availability of oxygen to the tissues in neonates, but this problem quickly decreases with age.

7. Because of their size, paediatric patients have a low total circulating blood volume. Any haemorrhage during surgery is serious and likely to lead to hypovolaemic shock. Therefore, blood loss needs to be minimised and hypovolaemia should always be treated. In addition, neonates have an increased tendency to bleeding disorders especially disseminated intravascular coagulation (D.I.C.) if they become hypothermic and this can further complicate the management of anaesthesia and surgery.

MANAGEMENT

Ideally, neonatal animals should be kept with their dam until anaesthesia is induced. If this is not possible, ensure that they do not become hypothermic, hypoglycaemic or dehydrated by keeping the ambient temperature high and avoiding a prolonged period of pre-operative starvation or water deprivation.

The animal should be weighed accurately and drugs diluted to avoid the risk of overdosage.

TECHNIQUE

Local Analgesia

The risk of producing toxic side effects with local anaesthetic agents is increased in paediatric patients. The safe maximum dose of lignocaine is only 5 – 10 mg/kg (¼ – ½ ml 2% solution) in an adult and it is easy to exceed this when infiltrating around a surgical site in a small puppy. The reduced ability of neonates to metabolise the drug will further reduce the safe maximum dose. Overdosage of local anaesthetic agents in very young animals, leads to profound bradycardia, cardiovascular collapse and sometimes seizures. These agents are therefore best avoided.

Premedication

In animals up to 4 weeks of age, premedication is not usually required. However, slightly older puppies, of the larger breeds, may need some sedation and in these cases, small doses of pethidine (1 mg/kg) can be helpful. The use of phenothiazines should be avoided if possible, but if a greater degree of sedation is required than is achieved with pethidine alone, only small doses of acepromazine should be used (0.01 – 0.02 mg/kg), since the duration of action of these drugs, including their cardiovascular effects, will be considerably prolonged in young animals.

Anticholinergic drugs may well be required in paediatric patients if drugs which produce bradycardia are used, since cardiac output is dependent on rate. But, it is best to use these drugs only if specifically required rather than routinely, since there is real danger of making bronchial secretions more viscid and, therefore, more prone to plug bronchioles in neonatal animals.

Induction

Inhalation agents administered via a mask are undoubtedly preferable to any intravenously or intramuscularly administered drug. Halothane or isoflurane are the agents of choice because of the relatively fast rate of induction and recovery achieved with these agents.

In larger, older puppies (12 weeks), where restraint is a problem, a small dose of propofol or methohexitone may be required, but only an amount sufficient drug to achieve light anaesthesia should be used, before deepening to the point of intubation by the use of an inhalational agent.

Maintenance

Inhalational agents (halothane or isoflurane) should be used to maintain anaesthesia and they should be delivered via apparatus which must be light, simple and have minimal deadspace. It must also allow easy access to the patient and permit I.P.P.V. if needed. If a mask is used, a high fresh gas flow will be required to prevent rebreathing. If the animal is intubated, care must be taken not to traumatise the larynx as laryngeal oedema may well occur post anaesthesia. Uncuffed tubes allow a greater diameter airway and soft tubes are preferable. The tube should be cut to an appropriate length so that it neither enters a bronchus nor protrudes beyond the mouth thereby increasing dead space.

A modified 'T' piece or a Bain coaxial breathing circuit should be used in order to minimise the work of breathing and to reduce dead space. There is a degree of heat and fluid loss which occurs through the respiratory tract when an unmodified Ayre's 'T' piece is used but this can be minimised by using the Jackson-Rees modification.

The carrier gas should comprise at least 50% oxygen since young animals have a much higher rate of oxygen consumption than adults.

Intravenous fluid administration should be carried out very cautiously since pups and kittens cannot tolerate over-infusion and are prone to develop pulmonary oedema. A paediatric burette should be used so that small volumes can be given accurately. Only that which has been lost should be replaced (evaporative losses generally average 5—10 ml/kg/hr of surgery). Blood loss in excess of 10% of total blood volume should be replaced on a volume for volume basis (in a 5 kg pup, a 10% blood loss = 40 ml). A glucose containing solution (e.g. a mixture of 5% dextrose and hartmann's) is useful as it will prevent the development of hypoglycaemia.

Muscle relaxants. Specific muscle relaxant drugs are not required since young animals have poorly developed musculature and should I.P.P.V. be required, control of the respiration is easily achieved by rhythmic manual compression of the rebreathing bag.

Monitoring

In young animals, the depth of anaesthesia can fluctuate quickly, so close monitoring is essential. An oesophageal stethoscope is invaluable since pulses may be difficult to find in tiny patients. Respiratory rates and mucous membrane colour must also be watched closely.

Young animals also lose heat rapidly so it is essential to monitor body temperature and to take steps to minimise losses (high ambient temperature, insulating blankets) and provide heat if necessary (heating pads).

Postoperative Care

Careful observation is essential. Delayed recovery, hypothermia, hypoglycaemia and respiratory depression are all too common in paediatric patients.
It is important to maintain body temperature and take steps to return the animal to normothermia as soon as possible. If recovery is delayed, these animals should be placed in a warm (T° 75—80° F) oxygen enriched atmosphere (an incubator is ideal) and also be given glucose intravenously if hypoglycaemia is suspected.

Pain relief should be provided by the judicious use of pethidine 1—2 mg/kg I/M.

FURTHER READING

HALL, L. W. (1972) Anaesthesia and euthanasia of neonatal and juvenile dogs and cats. *Vet Rec* **90,** 303-306.
ROBINSON, E. P. (1983) Anaesthesia of paediatric patients. *Comp. Cont. Ed. Vol 5,* 1004-1011.

CHAPTER 14

ANAESTHESIA IN HIGH RISK CASES

A. E. Waterman B.V.Sc., Ph.D., D.V.A., M.R.C.V.S.

GENERAL CONSIDERATIONS

It is clearly impossible to cover all the diverse conditions and circumstances under which anaesthesia may pose problems and to document in detail how each case should be managed. However, there are broad principles which can be followed.

Healthy animals can withstand the insult of anaesthesia very well; however, the critically ill patient will lack normal homeostatic balances and is less able to compensate for any cardiovascular, respiratory or metabolic insult.

It is important to determine whether anaesthesia is absolutely essential or whether the procedure could be postponed until the patient is stabilised. Finally, one must choose the technique least harmful to the animal.

PRE-ANAESTHETIC PREPARATION

A full and thorough examination is essential in all except the most extreme emergencies such as respiratory arrest or severe haemorrhage. In these situations, immediate resuscitation is obviously the first priority; once the animal is stabilised, a thorough evaluation can be performed.

This includes:-

1. **History.**

   A careful evaluation of past clinical history and the current problem should be made. In trauma cases, it is useful to know whether the animal suffered abdominal or thoracic trauma and whether it lost consciousness. Non-trauma cases admitted as emergencies are generally severely dehydrated and in circulatory shock. Examples of these cases include gastric torsion and dilation, acute intestinal obstruction, urinary tract obstruction and severe pyometritis. It is vital to obtain a detailed description of the nature, duration and severity of signs, so that some estimate of the nature and size of the fluid deficit may be obtained (see chapter 15).

2. Examination.

The animal should be examined systematically, using a check list so that nothing is overlooked and any abnormalities found should be noted.

CHECK:

a.	general appearance	
b.	cardiovascular system	capilliary refill time (C.R.T.) pulse rate and volume heart rate and rhythm
c.	respiratory system	upper airways thoracic movements auscultation colour of mucous membranes
d.	integument	skin pliability
e.	gastro-intestinal tract	abdominal palpation pain or fluid thrill
f.	urinary tract	
g.	central nervous system	
h.	visual and auditory systems	
i.	musculoskeletal system	

3. Emergency Treatment.

It is essential to stabilise the animal before performing major procedures.

a. establish an airway and give oxygen if needed: either by endotracheal intubation or tracheotomy (sedation may be required for tracheotomy).

b. cover any open chest wounds in trauma cases

c. drain any large pneumothorax

d. set up an I/V infusion and treat shock

e. relieve gastric tympany if present, by tube decompression or trocarisation

4. Laboratory Evaluation.

Blood should be obtained for evaluation. Even if therapy must begin before the results are known, at least baseline data will be available so that treatment can be monitored logically.

a.	haematology	packed cell volume (P.C.V.) white blood cell count (W.B.C.)
b.	biochemistry	blood urea total plasma proteins serum amylase (if pancreatitis suspected) blood electrolytes (especially K^+)

c. blood gases and acid-base balance information is useful but beyond the scope of most practice laboratories

5. Radiography.

There is almost no situation where anaesthesia and surgery need to proceed without first obtaining radiographic assistance in determining the extent of the problem. Radiography is essential in trauma cases and also extremely valuable in assessing gastro-intestinal problems.

PREMEDICATION

The dosages of all C.N.S. depressant drugs should be reduced in critically ill animals.

The phenothiazines can be useful in that they will sedate the animal but they cause marked hypotension and hypothermia and their effects are likely to be enhanced and prolonged in sick animals, especially those suffering from hypovolaemia, unless intravenous fluids are given first. If they are used, the dose rate should be reduced by 50% (i.e. to 0.025—0.05 mg/kg).

Xylazine has marked cardiovascular and respiratory effects which make it dangerous in critically ill patients and its use is not recommended in these cases. The marked respiratory and cardiovascular depression produced by medetomidine will also preclude the safe use of this drug in high risk cases. Benzodiazepines such as diazepam or midazolam are not very effective sedatives in healthy dogs and cats, but in very ill animals their minimal cardiovascular and respiratory depressant effects make them valuable agents, especially in combination with analgesic drugs (diazepam dose 0.2—0.5 mg/kg I/M or I/V).

Analgesics such as pethidine or morphine are extremely useful in high risk cases. These drugs have little effect on the cardiovascular system (although the more potent fentanyl or alfentanyl may produce a bradycardia) and although there is a theoretical risk of producing respiratory depression, this is much less common in animals which are in pain. They have the added advantage that they also have sedative effects and they are often all that is necessary to provide sedation in these cases. The availability of specific antagonists such as naloxone also enhances the safety of these drugs.

	I/M Dose:
Morphine	Dogs: 0.1—0.2 mg/kg
Pethidine	Dogs: 1—3 mg/kg
	Cats: 3.5 mg/kg

Anticholinergic drugs are indicated if vagotonic agents are given or if acid base imbalances, which predispose to bradycardia, are present, since critically ill patients are less able to cope with periods of bradycardia and hypotension.

INDUCTION OF GENERAL ANAESTHESIA

It is difficult to advocate any one particular technique since circumstances and facilities vary.

I/V. Short acting drugs should be chosen and the anaesthetist must be prepared to reduce dose rates considerably. The agent should be given slowly and to effect. In dogs, a 'sleep' dose of thiopentone (5—6 mg/kg) or propofol (3—4 mg/kg) is usually all that is required.

Inhalation. In really sick animals, anaesthesia may be easily achieved by the administration of halothane (or isoflurane) in O_2 or O_2 and N_2O, but there are some circumstances (e.g. respiratory problems) when anaesthesia needs to be induced very quickly and then an I/V agent must be used.

In cats the steroid anaesthetic 'Saffan' may be used as an alternative to thiopentone or 'propofol' for the induction of anaesthesia.

Ketamine is a dissociative anaesthetic agent which, unlike any other anaesthetic agent, produces stimulation of the cardiovascular system. When used alone it produces marked rigidity, but when combined with diazepam, it produces a state resembling anaesthesia and it has been advocated by some for the induction of anaesthesia in poor risk cases. However, since the drug relies on hepatic metabolism and renal excretion for cessation of its action, it should be used with extreme caution in animals with dysfunction of these organs (which would include animals suffering from hypovolaemic shock).

MAINTENANCE OF ANAESTHESIA

Anaesthesia should be maintained with a volatile agent (usually halothane O_2 with or without N_2O).

One must aim to provide at least 30% and preferably 40—50% inspired O_2.

It is vital to have full control of the airway, therefore endotracheal intubation is essential and hypoventilation must be avoided.

In order to keep the plane of anaesthesia as light as possible, a calibrated vaporiser is an advantage.

If facilities are available, there is much to commend the use of a technique utilising IPPV, a muscle relaxant and a very low inspired percentage of a volatile agent and/or an analgesic. However, if the animal is severely hypovolaemic, venous return may be impaired by a prolonged application of positive pressure to the thorax.

MONITORING

Cardiovascular system. Heart rate should be monitored (normal range 70—180). Critically ill patients are likely to have lowered cardiac reserves and therefore heart rate and rhythm and blood pressure may be more variable as the body is less able to adapt to changes, making the onset of arrhythmias and shock more likely.

Fluid Balance. An I/V infusion should be set up and fluid losses and urinary output monitored; over-infusion should be avoided. Hypovolaemic shock should be treated appropriately.

Respiratory System. Rate and depth of respiration should be monitored. Hypoventilation, which will lead to hypercarbia and hypoxia, should be avoided. The colour of mucous membranes should be monitored. If they become blue or bright red, ventilation should be assisted.

Thermoregulation. Rectal temperature and the core-peripheral temperature gradient, which tends to widen in shock as peripheral vasoconstriction occurs, should be monitored. Hypothermia should be avoided.

Depth of Anaesthesia. Anaesthesia should be kept as light as possible. Experience has shown that less drug is required to produce a given depth of anaesthesia in sick, compared to fit, animals. Jaw tone can be quite useful as a guide to the depth of anaesthesia in these cases; if the jaw is slack, anaesthesia is probably too deep.

POST-OPERATIVE PERIOD

Monitoring of vital functions must continue in the post-operative period in these patients for at least 12—24 hours. Body temperature, fluid input, urinary output, colour of mucous membranes and C.R.T. should be recorded as well as heart and respiratory rates.

Problems which are commonly encountered are hypothermia, hypoxia and fluid imbalances, and appropriate remedial measures must be instituted.

Provision of adequate pain relief is also essential. Pethidine at a dose rate of 2.0—3.5 mg/kg will provide effective analgesia for 2—3 hours and, should the animal become restless, diazepam (0.25 mg/kg) may also be administered.

It is also useful to maintain an indwelling I/V catheter for at least 24 hours.

CASE EXAMPLES — SPECIAL PROBLEMS

Head Trauma

A rise in intracranial pressure should be avoided by hyperventilating and avoiding the use of vasodilators.

IPPV with O_2 and N_2O with or without a low percentage of a volatile agent is preferred.
A short acting narcotic can be given.

Non-specific Trauma

It is more important to treat pain rather than to aim at sedation.

S/C or I/M injection should be avoided in shock as absorption will be poor.

A full stomach will predispose to vomiting on induction.

Gastric Dilation/Torsion

Hypovolaemic shock and metabolic acidosis must be corrected.

Severe arrhythmias may develop, which may need treating.

Maximal ventilatory support should be provided.

Urethral obstruction in cats

Cats will be dehydrated, uraemic, acidotic and hyperkalaemic.

Halothane may well precipitate severe cardiac dysrhythmias, even to the extent of precipitating a cardiac arrest.

Xylazine also will potentiate dysrhythmias and have a prolonged duration of action in these cases.

Ketamine also will have a prolonged duration of action.

A short-acting drug such as 'Saffan' or propofol is best used if anaesthesia is essential for relieving the obstruction, but the animal should be stabilised before embarking on major surgery.

Rupture of the urinary bladder

Animals which sustain rupture of the urinary bladder or urethra quickly develop hyperkalaemia, metabolic acidosis, uraemia and dehydration. It is these disturbances which ultimately prove fatal.

There can be no justification for attempting corrective surgery before the animal is stabilised, since immediate anaesthesia carries a high and unacceptable risk of provoking cardiac dysrhythmias, severe cardiovascular collapse and even cardiac arrest.

The first line of treatment must be correction of the metabolic derangements, especially the hyperkalaemia and acidosis. This may be achieved by a combination of I/V fluids, additional bicarbonate therapy and urinary catheterisation and/or paracentesis as appropriate. Only when the metabolic disturbances have been corrected should anaesthesia and surgery be contemplated.

Intestinal obstruction

These animals die of dehydration, hypovolaemic shock and the metabolic consequences of the obstruction. The first priority must be to restore the fluid and electrolyte deficits rather than to embark on immediate surgery.

CHAPTER 15

FLUID THERAPY

J. C. Brearley M.A., Vet. M.B., D.V.A., M.R.C.V.S.

Rule of thumb:-

REPLACE LIKE WITH LIKE, RATE WITH RATE, VOLUME WITH VOLUME

INDICATIONS FOR FLUID THERAPY

Restoration and maintenance of fluid and electrolyte balance.

To assist the promotion of diuresis.

To provide a vehicle for dialysis.

(Alimentation).

(To maintain an 'open vein').

This chapter will concentrate on the first of these as this is the most common indication encountered in connection with anaesthesia. In this role therapy, for the most part, is not curative but aims at correcting a fluid imbalance which may have arisen from a variety of causes. Persistent imbalance will lead to the development of irreversible shock, which may be defined as 'a clinical condition characterised by signs and symptoms which arise when cardiac output is insufficient to fill the arterial tree with blood under sufficient pressure to provide organs and tissues with adequate blood flow' (Simeone 1964). Unless the underlying cause is determined and treated, the imbalance will recur and shock develop. Whatever the aetiology, a severe fluid deficit can be life-threatening and requires prompt attention.

To enable an informed approach to fluid therapy, some understanding of normal fluid distribution and composition is required in conjunction with an appreciation of the constituents of available replacement fluids, (Fig. 15.1 and Table 15.1.)

Figure 15.1
Summary of Fluid Distribution within the Body and Daily Requirements

DISTRIBUTION.

Total body water   Adult dog c.60% body weight, at birth 84%

⅓ extracellular (ECF) made up of:

interstitial and transcellular ¾
intravascular ¼
most available to manipulation

⅔ intracellular (ICF)

Blood volume   88 ml/kg body weight.
Higher in the young, lower in the obese.

DAILY REQUIREMENTS IN A NORMAL ANIMAL IN BALANCE

To replace water   Insensible (inevitable) loss   minus 20 ml/kg day
Regulatable loss (urinary)   minus 20 ml/kg/day
vis 40 ml/kg/day is a rough guide for maintenance.

To replace sodium   1mEq/kg/day
potassium   2mEq/kg/day

Table 15.1
Composition of some Crystalloid Fluids and some Endogenous Fluids in Dogs

FLUID	SODIUM (mmol/l)	CHLORIDE (mmol/l)	POTASSIUM (mmol/l)	CALCIUM (mmol/l)	GLUCOSE (mmol/l)
ICF	10	2	150		
plasma	142-150	105-120	3.7-5	2.2-2.7	3.4-5.3
saline (0.9%)	154	154	—	—	—
N/5 saline + 4.3% dextrose	31	31	—	—	195
hartmann's	140	100	5	trace	—
5% dextrose	—	—	—	—	227

DIAGNOSIS OF FLUID IMBALANCES

HISTORY

This should pay particular reference to fluid input, output and distribution. Although fluid intake is notoriously difficult to estimate from a history, questions relating to the volume of the drinking bowl and the frequency of refilling which will help. Duration of illness, urination history, frequency of vomiting and/or diarrhoea, may give an indication of fluid output. Evaporative losses, e.g. by panting, pyrexia, open wounds or burns, are often overlooked as a source of fluid loss by evaporation but may be of great importance. Obvious trauma or blood loss will be presenting signs rather than being ascertained from a history.

CLINICAL EXAMINATION

The systems reflecting fluid imbalance in particular are the cardiovascular, respiratory and gastrointestinal. However, the whole body will be affected as roughly 60% of the total body weight is made up of water. Certain clinical signs may suggest specific imbalances (Table 15.2a) and may give a rough guide to the degree of dehydration (Table 15.2b).

Table 15.2a
Imbalances and Clinical Signs

TYPE OF LOSS	TYPICAL CLINICAL SIGNS AND HISTORY
Water loss	Thirst, dry mucous membranes, reduced urine output, weakness and lethargy. Animal does not look very ill until large deficit present. Arises from decreased intake and increased insensible losses, e.g. prolonged panting, polyuria, pyrexia.
Mixed water and electrolyte	Decreased skin turgor, poor pulse, cold extremities. Animal looks ill. This is the commonest type of deficit. Occurs with vomiting and diarrhoea.
Acid-base imbalance	Generally diagnosed from history and predictions from existing clinical condition. Gastric vomiting is associated with metabolic alkalosis, duodenal vomiting (i.e. bile stained vomitus), metabolic acidosis. Acidosis is also common with diarrhoea, diabetes mellitus and 'shock' with lactic acid accumulation
Blood loss	This may be acute or chronic, external or internal. Mucous membranes pale, cold extremities, poor pulse. External loss will be obvious by the presence of bleeding points but internal haemorrhage may be more difficult to differentiate from shock than from other causes. However, the initial treatment is the same, i.e. plasma volume expansion. This will allow time to obtain a haematocrit or haemoglobin which will aid the diagnosis.

Table 15.2b
Percentage Dehydration and Clinical Signs

% DEHYDRATION	CLINICAL SIGNS
< 5% slight	Not detectable
5–6 % mild	Slightly decreased skin turgor
6–8% mild	Delay in skin fold return, slight increase in capillary refill time. Eyes may be slightly sunken. May have dry mucous membranes.
10–12 % moderate	Tenting of skin. Increased capillary refill time, sunken eyes, dry mucous membranes, tachycardia ± cold extremities, weak pulse, (possible signs of shock)
12–15 % severe	Shock ± death

CLINICAL MEASUREMENTS

Capillary refill time.

This is normally less than 2 seconds. A longer time suggests reduced peripheral perfusion either due to frank fluid loss or to inappropriate distribution i.e. shock.

Mucous membrane colour.

This is normally salmon pink. Variations in colour ranging from parchment (suggestive of vasoconstriction or anaemia) to purple (which may indicate toxaemia) are clinically useful.

Peripheral pulse.

For example, labial, lingual, dorsal pedal or palmar metacarpal. The presence of pulses indicates that the arterial blood pressure is adequate to maintain blood flow to peripheral tissues and hence to vital organs. Conversely, absence of these pulses indicates low arterial blood pressure.

Skin turgor.

If the skin is pinched into a fold, the fold should immediately disappear on release. Failure to do so may indicate a state of dehydration, but can also occur in cachetic patients or Cushingoid animals. Conversely fat, dehydrated animals, will less readily show decreased skin turgor.

Urinary output.

This is an important means of determining fluid status, when renal function is normal, and can be used as a monitoring aid during anaesthesia. The bladder is catheterised and emptied. A cheap means of collecting and measuring the volume of urine is to connect the catheter to one end of an intravenous extension tubing and an empty fluid administration bag to the other end. A production rate of at least 1 ml/kg/hr is considered to indicate adequate renal perfusion and renal function. Any rate less than this is a positive indication for monitored fluid therapy.

Central venous pressure (CVP).

This provides information about venous volume and the efficiency of the pumping capacity of the right side of the heart. A long jugular catheter is aseptically inserted into the anterior vena cava. The distal end is attached to a fluid manometer and fluid reservoir via a giving set. The zero point of the manometer is set level with the right atrium, although the sternum is taken as the external reference point. Measurement is made by filling the manometer column from the reservoir and then opening the column to the intravenous line, whilst stopping the flow from the reservoir. The manometer fluid column will fall rapidly initially. The central venous pressure is equal to the height of the column once this rapid fall ceases. This intravenous line can also be used to give crystalloid fluids from the reservoir. The normal CVP in dogs is 3—7 cms water irrespective of the position of the animal. A low CVP is indicative of inadequate circulating blood volume and replacement should be given. A high CVP indicates either fluid overload or right sided heart failure and fluid infusions should be stopped immediately. Peripheral venous pressure can be similarly measured with a catheter in a peripheral vein but is only of use as an aid to monitoring fluid administration; it should not be used as a diagnostic aid.

Laboratory measurements.

For example, haematocrit, haemoglobin, sodium, potassium, urea, creatinine and total plasma protein. An isolated value is of limited use in the diagnosis of fluid imbalances but serial estimations during therapy will indicate the success or otherwise of the therapy. During dehydration, the concentration of all these parameters will rise, but high concentrations can occur in other conditions unrelated to fluid balance. If the animal is not anaemic, or polycythaemic, a raised haematocrit and total plasma protein can be used to give an indication of the size of the fluid deficit.

Arterial blood pressure.

Direct arterial blood pressure measurement requires arterial catheterisation and an anaeroid manometer or electronic pressure transducer. Indirect measurement techniques include doppler and infrared photocells. Neither technique is widely used outside specialist centres probably due to expense and unfamiliarity, but it provides the most useful information of all the clinical measurements mentioned and provides a sensitive intra-operative assessment aid of depth of anaesthesia and fluid balance.

ROUTES OF FLUID REPLACEMENT

Oral.

If the animal is suffering mild to moderate water and/or electrolyte loss, is conscious and there is no reason why gut absorption cannot take place (e.g. intestinal obstruction), then the oral route is the method of choice. It allows self regulation of fluid and electrolyte absorption and so overload is avoided. If the animal is unable to either lap or swallow, a nasogastric or pharyngostomy tube should be considered.

Subcutaneous.

This is an unsuitable route of administration for all but very mildly dehydrated animals which would be better receiving oral fluids where possible. Blood flow to subcutaneous tissues is poor in a normally hydrated animal; in a dehydrated animal, compensatory mechanisms will reduce perfusion further and thus there will be little absorption from this site.

Intravenous administration.

This is the method of choice in animals in which the oral route is unavailable or contraindicated. A plastic intravenous catheter, well secured to the skin either by sutures or by tape, is least likely to be dislodged, thereby reducing the risk of accidental extravascular administration. In moderately dehydrated animals, a limb vein may be used, but in severely collapsed animals, a jugular cut-down may be required to allow placement of the intravenous catheter. Intravenous catheters should be replaced every 48 hours and when not in use, flushed with heparinized saline. This is the only route by which blood, colloids, hypertonic fluids and parenteral nutrition may be given.

Intraperitoneal administration.

For use in animals which are too small to allow secure placement of an intravenous catheter, e.g. neonates, small rodents. This route has the advantage of a potentially large surface area of absorption, i.e. the intestines; the disadvantages are that there is a risk of visceral puncture, leading to haemorrhage or peritonitis and there is little control over the amount of fluid absorbed. Intraperitoneal fluids may also be used to lavage the abdominal cavity, either in the case of peritonitis, or as a means of dialysis in uraemic animals.

TYPES OF FLUID

Blood

This is used in cases of severe haemorrhage or anaemia. It must be collected aseptically into anticoagulant (e.g. citrate) and only used with a filter in the giving line. Whole blood has a limited shelf-life of up to 4 weeks if kept at +4°C in a refrigerator. Cross matching should be undertaken if the recipient has had previous a transfusion.

Plasma

This is used in conditions of hypoproteinaemia (e.g. liver disease), hypoglobulinaemia (e.g. premature neonates), or conditions in which clotting factors may be deficient (e.g. prolonged bleeding or disseminated intravascular coagulation), where red blood cells are not deficient. Plasma is collected from centrifuged anticoagulated whole blood. There are similar problems of sterility as with whole blood. When rapidly frozen and stored at −20°C, it will keep for up to a year.

Colloids

Plasma volume replacers (e.g. gelatin based substitutes — 'Haemacel', 'Gelofusin'), are used to replace fluid deficits in the circulating blood volume without drawing fluid in from the extracellular fluid volume. They are useful in combination with crystalloids in conditions of severe dehydration of mixed origin with a degree of circulatory collapse or to maintain arterial blood pressure in shock or haemorrhage.

Plasma volume expanders (e.g. dextran 70 — 'Macrodex') expand the plasma volume by oncotically drawing fluid from the extravascular, extracellular space into the circulation, thus increasing the plasma volume by an amount greater than the volume of exogenous fluid infused. They are used in cases of circulatory collapse with a relatively normal extravascular hydration, e.g. severe haemorrhage, and can interfere with blood coagulation mechanisms and cross-matching if given in large volumes. All colloids should be used with caution in conditions where capillary leakage is likely, e.g. toxaemic shock, as they will not be resorbed from the extravascular space when the animal's condition improves and the integrity of the capillaries is restored.

Crystalloids

These are composed of water, electrolytes and/or dextrose. They can be used in cases of circulatory collapse to improve the plasma volume, but larger volumes must be given to achieve the same effect as colloids, as they will readily move from the intravascular volume into the extravascular space. This gives the disadvantage of increased risk of pulmonary oedema, but the advantage of more readily re-entering the vascular space if oedema does occur. The indications for the use of crystalloids vary with the composition of the fluid but, in general, they are used as routine maintenance and replacement fluids.

REPLACE LIKE WITH LIKE

If abnormal losses occur, restitution must be made by administering water, electrolytes or blood constituents in the proportion that they are lost. First, the nature of the losses must be ascertained. This is done by obtaining a detailed history. A careful clinical examination will provide further information. Laboratory tests are perhaps of more use in this context than determining the volume of losses or the rate by which they occurred. Blood losses will be reflected in a low haematocrit and/or haemoglobin, with normal or low total plasma proteins. Plasma electrolytes remain remarkably stable in the main, due to compensatory mechanisms; potassium is the least compensated in such circumstances. Urea and creatinine will increase in dehydration due to pre-renal failure.

Additives to crystalloid solutions include potassium chloride (should be given with care and serum potassium monitoring), sodium bicarbonate in metabolic acidosis, glucose in animals in which oral intake is contraindicated for a prolonged period (but intravenous glucose alone will not meet total energy requirements as high concentrations will cause osmotic diuresis by glycosuria).

Bicarbonate varies in plasma with the plasma pH and carbon dioxide tension: an average value is around 25 mmol/L. The only commonly used replacement fluid which contains a bicarbonate precursor, is hartmann's solution. Sodium bicarbonate solution is available in various strengths and this may be used to correct metabolic acidosis but is not a replacement fluid in the accepted sense of the term.

An 8.4% sodium bicarbonate solution contains 1 mEq/ml. Where acidosis is suspected but cannot be measured, the administration of 1 mEq/kg is considered safe. Over-enthusiastic use of sodium bicarbonate is the commonest cause of metabolic alkalosis, which may be more harmful than the original acidosis as it reduces oxygen availability to tissues and produces respiratory depression.

Table 15.3
Conditions, Depletions and Replacements

CONDITION	DEPLETIONS	REPLACEMENT FLUID
Severe bleeding > 10% total blood volume	whole blood (RBC, plasma)	whole blood if available or plasma volume expander, with oxygen supplementation
Moderate bleeding < 10% total blood volume	whole blood	plasma volume replacer or expander sufficient
Mild bleeding	whole blood	Hartmann's or colloids
Gastric vomiting	H^+, Na^+, Cl^-, water	Normal saline (0.9%) (+ KCl 10–20 mmol/l if prolonged)
Duodenal vomiting	mixed depletion	Hartmann's
Diarrhoea	Na^+, Cl^-, HCO_3^-, K^+, water	Hartmann's (+ HCO_3 2–3 mmol/l + KCl 10–20 mmol/l if severe or prolonged)
Intestinal obstruction	severe, mixed depletion	Hartmann's (+ plasma volume expander if in hypovolaemic shock)
Maintenance	none	N/5 saline + 4.3% dextrose
Reduced intake e.g. reduced awareness anaesthesia	water	5% dextrose or N/5 saline + 4.3% dextrose
Ruptured bladder	retention of K^+, H^+	0.9% saline or N/5 saline + 4.3% dextrose (HCO_3 2–3 mmol/kg added to reduce acidosis and drive K^+ ions into the cells).

REPLACE RATE WITH RATE

Due to the homoeostatic mechanisms, if depletions take place over a long period of time, the body will compensate to maintain function of vital organs. (e.g. by antidiuretic hormone and aldosterone release, gastrointestinal tract absorption and increased intake and oxidation of body tissues to produce metabolic water.) The classical example of this is the polyuria-induced polydipsia of diabetes. Problems arise when something interferes with the compensatory mechanism, (e.g. enforced reduced intake or reduced sympathomimetic activity as in anaesthesia) when an acute depletion occurs on top of a chronic situation, a depletion occurs so rapidly that the body cannot compensate or the depletion is so great that the body can no longer compensate.

As a general rule, depletions that take place rapidly should be replaced rapidly, and vice versa. Any circulatory deficit can be replaced rapidly as long as the heart is not overloaded. Up to 90 ml/kg/hour, or one blood volume, may be given in hypovolaemic shock if cardiovascular and renal function is normal and central venous pressure and urine output is monitored. However, a rate of 10 ml/kg/hour should be regarded as a maximum if the infusion is to be given for more than a few minutes at this rate. Extravascular depletions need to be repaired more slowly as transfer out of the vascular space must occur. Thus, severe depletions may take up to 48 hours to repair, during which time ongoing losses must also be allowed for and maintenance requirements met.

The administration rate should be converted from ml/kg/hour to drops/minute, to allow ease of administration. thus:-

$$\frac{\text{drops/ml delivered by the infusion set}}{60} \times \text{ml/kg/hour} \times \text{body weight (kg)} = \textbf{drops/minute}$$

Most infusion sets deliver 15 drops / ml, but this should be checked on the packaging of the set before the infusion is started. Burettes or pediatric giving sets are very useful, if not essential, in tiny animals, to avoid fluid overload. These deliver 50 drops/ml.

REPLACE VOLUME WITH VOLUME

This is where knowledge of distribution of fluid within the body is important. If a deficit occurs over a few days, the loss will be from the whole body. Thus, the water deficit will be divided into one third extracellular and two thirds intracellular. Of the ECF, one quarter will be plasma deficit and the rest will come from the interstitial volume. As mentioned above, the plasma deficit can be replaced rapidly but the remaining deficit should be administered over 24 — 48 hours, in addition to allowing for the maintenance requirements.

Various means of estimating the size of the imbalance have been advocated:

Calculation from history:-

Losses

Allow for insensible losses of 20 ml/kg/day of reduced intake and urinary losses of 20 ml/kg/day through normal urination. Add 1 ml/kg for losses through vomitus and some estimation of the volume of any diarrhoea or lost blood plus some allowance for any panting and pyrexia.

Intake

Intake will equal the volume of drinking bowl, multiplied by the number of times the bowl is filled daily.

If the intake and the losses are equal then the patient is in fluid balance.

Example

A two year old dog weighing 10 kg has been ill for 2 days, vomiting for the last 24 hours (5 times). During the last 12 hours it has passed watery diarrhoea 3 times (approximately 50 ml each time). It has not urinated for the past day.

Insensible losses at 20 ml/kg/day for 2 days	400 ml
One day normal urination at 20/ml/kg/day	200 ml
Faecal losses 3 x 50 ml	150 ml
Losses in vomitus x 5 at 1 ml/kg/vomit	50 ml
Total water deficit	1000 ml
ECF (⅓ TWD)	333 ml
Plasma deficit (¼ ECF)	83 ml
(Total blood volume at 88 ml/kg	880 ml)

Approximately 1/10th of the circulating blood volume has been lost and therefore this could be replaced rapidly by a colloid and the remaining deficit by hartmann's solution over the next 24 hours. Alternatively, the whole deficit could be replaced by hartmann's over 24 hours if the dog is not collapsed.

Calculation from haematocrit

For every 1% rise in haematocrit above 45%, allow 10 ml/kg body weight.

NOTE: fit animals and certain breeds of dogs may have an elevated haematocrit normally, so ideally a pre-haemorrhage haematocrit should be known.

Calculation from weight changes

This requires knowledge of the animal's normal weight. Any abrupt changes in weight will be due to either gut filling or water balance. In an animal with no intake, it will obviously be due to changes in water content of the body.

(1 litre of water weighs 1 kg).

Calculation of surgical losses

Intra-operative blood losses may be estimated either by multiplying the number of used swabs of known capacity (ml) by the known capacity, or by weighing the used swabs of known unused weight (assuming 1g blood = 1ml blood volume) and adding half the above amount for spillage not swabbed and the volume of blood collected by suction.

This should be replaced by:-

A crystalloid if the loss is less than 10% of the total blood volume.

A colloid if the loss is greater than 10% of the total blood volume.

Whole blood if the loss is more than 15% of the total blood volume.

Allowance must be made for inevitable losses still occurring whilst the animal is unable to ingest fluids either due to absence of fluid in the environment (e.g., removal of water for up to 12 hours preoperatively), unconsciousness due to anaesthesia or reduced awareness due to heavy sedation.

A chart should be made of fluid balance, recording all fluid administered and all losses, (e.g. blood loss, urination, faecal output, vomitus). This should also include daily weighing of the animal as this will provide the most accurate estimate of fluid balance. As an aid to giving fluids, the volume to be given in one hour should be marked on the infusion bag.

FURTHER READING

ALLEN, D. (1986). Crystalloids versus colloids. *Am. J. Vet. Res.* **47** (8) : 1751-1755.
CROWE, D. T. (1986). Clinical use of an indwelling nasogastric tube for enteral nutrition and fluid therapy in the dog and cat. *J. Am. Anim. Hosp. Ass.* **22**, 675-682.
DESSIRIS, A. (1987). Peripheral venous pressure as a guide for fluid administration in hypovolaemic dogs. *Zblt. Vet. Med. A* **34** (9) : 690-698.
FALER, K. and FALER, K. (1985). Fluid therapy in large and small animals. *Mod. vet. Pract.* **66** : 635-639.
FETTMAN, M. J. (1985). Hypertonic crystalloid solutions for treating hemorrhagic shock. *Comp. Cont. Education,* **7**, (11) ; 915-920.
GOLDSTON, R. T., WILKES, R. D. and SEYBOLD, I. (1983). Water electrolyte and acid/base balance. *Vet. Med./small Anim. Clin.* (January 1983) : 31-35.
HALL, L. W. (1980). Preliminary investigations of the effects of injury on the body fluids of cats and dogs. *J. small Anim. Pract.* **21**, : 679-689.
HASKINS, S. C. (1984). Fluid and electrolyte therapy. *Comp. Cont. Education* **6** (3) : 244-254.
MICHELL, A. R. (1983). Understanding fluid therapy. *Irish Veterinary Journal* **37**, : 94-103.
MICHELL, A. R. (1988 in prep.). *Veterinary Fluid Therapy.* Blackwell Scientific Publications, Oxford.
SCHAER, M. (1982). (Editor). Fluid and electrolyte balance. *The Veterinary Clinics of North America : Small Animal Practice,* **12**, (3) whole issue. W. B. Saunders Company, Philadelphia.
WATERMAN, A, E. (1984). Practical fluid therapy for small animals. In *Practice,* Sept 1984, 143-150.
WATERMAN, A. E. (1979). Body Fluids. In: *Canine Medicine and Therapeutics.* Ed. E. A. Chandler et al., Ch. 11, 246-264. Blackwell Scientific Publications, Oxford.

CHAPTER 16
ANAESTHETIC ACCIDENTS AND EMERGENCIES

D. L. S. Richards B.Vet.Sc., D.V.A., M.R.C.V.S.

INTRODUCTION

Many anaesthetic accidents and emergencies can be prevented with careful pre-operative preparation and good anaesthetic management. However, accidents will happen and it is wise to be prepared for them.

A kit containing the items which may be needed during an emergency should be available (Table 1, page 136) together with a chart displaying the indications and dosages of the drugs which are commonly used during a resuscitation attempt (Table 2, page 137). It is important that staff are acquainted with these so that they may be used efficiently in an emergency situation.

The outcome of an emergency depends on recognising a problem rapidly, diagnosing the cause quickly and applying the appropriate remedy promptly. The following has been compiled with these objectives in mind.

RESPIRATORY PROBLEMS

RESPIRATORY OBSTRUCTION

Prevention of the free flow of gas within the airways, leading to hypoxia and hypercarbia.

Signs

1. Dyspnoea:- exaggerated inspiratory effort often accompanied by inward movement of the chest wall.
2. Respiratory insufficiency or arrest, (especially when anaesthetised).
3. 'Snoring' associated with partial obstruction.
4. Coughing or cyanosis (not seen with oxygen administration).

Causes

1. Soft tissue entrapment such as the tongue, soft palate or everted ventricles (brachycephalics).
2. Pathology such as laryngeal paralysis, laryngeal oedema, laryngospasm, collapsing trachea or bronchospasm.
3. 'Foreign' material such as blood clots, mucus, saliva, vomitus, teeth, calculi.
4. Mechanical obstruction such as constrictive bandages, kinked endotracheal tubes, an over-inflated cuff, high circuit resistance or endobronchial intubation.

Management

1. With an endotracheal tube already in place.
   a. Extend the head and neck.
   b. Check patency of the endotracheal tube; deflate and reinflate its cuff.
   c. Examine and if necessary, change the anaesthetic circuit.
   d. Reintubate the trachea.
2. Without an endotracheal tube in place.
   a. Extend the head and neck, pull the tongue forward and remove any bandages which may be causing obstruction.
   b. Examine the mouth and pharynx; remove any foreign material by suction or swabbing.
   c. Intubate the trachea. General anaesthesia may be needed. If laryngospasm is present use local anaesthetics or muscle relaxants to overcome it.
   d. Tracheotomy is not frequently necessary, but can be life saving in a case of laryngeal oedema. A 10–14 g needle or cannula, inserted between two tracheal rings, serves as a temporary measure. A tracheotomy is usually performed by cutting a tracheal ring longitudinally and inserting an endotracheal tube or special tracheotomy tube.
3. Special circumstances.
   a. In laryngeal oedema, corticosteroids may be needed.
   b. In bronchospasm — aminophylline, diprophylline or etamiphylline (all 5 mg/kg I/V); pethidine (2 mg/kg I/V); isoprenaline infusion (0.2 mg in 500 mls NaCl I/V to effect), may be given.

VENTILATORY INADEQUACY, APNOEA AND RESPIRATORY ARREST

When ventilation is inadequate to meet the body's metabolic needs.

Signs

1. Absence of respiration, (if temporary: apnoea; if persistent: respiratory arrest).
2. Reduced minute ventilation, usually seen as reduced tidal volume with increased, decreased or normal respiratory rates.
3. Cyanosis (if oxygen is not being used), tachycardia or cardiac arrhythmias may be seen.

Causes

1. Anaesthetic overdosage, especially with barbiturates, inhalants, opioids.
2. Hyperventilation leading to carbon dioxide washout.
3. Muscle relaxants.
4. Respiratory obstruction.
5. Reflex apnoea caused by, for instance, irritating vapours (ether), visceral traction or endotracheal intubation.
6. Pleural or pulmonary pathology e.g. pneumothorax, diaphragmatic hernia or pulmonary oedema.

Management

1. Stop anaesthetic administration.
2. Check that a pulse is present.
3. Establish a patent airway.
4. Ventilate the lungs using either an anaesthetic circuit (100% O_2), an Ambu bag (21% O_2) or the anaesthetist's own expirate (16% O_2). Administer 3–4 breaths rapidly followed by 6–12 breaths per minute until animal shows signs of maintaining its own ventilation.
5. Barbiturate apnoea following I/V thiopentone or methohexitone may last up to 5 minutes. Ventilate slowly (6 breaths per minute) to avoid hypocarbia.

6. Opioids can be antagonised using naloxone (10–20 ug/kg I/V) but this also antagonises analgesia. Diprenorphrine ('Small Animal Revivon') is the recommended antagonist for etorphine ('Small Animal Immobilon').

7. Medetomidine has a specific antagonist (atipamezole); other alpha-two antagonists (yohimbine, tolazoline, idazoxan) are experimental at present.

8. Non depolarising muscle relaxants can be antagonised using neostigmine (0.05 mg/kg I/V) preceded by atropine (0.04 mg/kg I/V).

9. Analeptics are not usually indicated. Doxapram (1.1 mg/kg I/V or sub-lingual) is useful in newborn puppies or kittens where endotracheal intubation is difficult to perform and ventilatory support impossible.

CARDIOVASCULAR PROBLEMS

HYPOTENSION

Reduced blood pressure resulting in poor organ perfusion.

Signs

1. A weak or imperceptible peripheral pulse.
2. (Usually) a prolonged capilliary refill time and pale mucous membranes.
3. (Usually) an elevated heart rate.
4. (Usually) congested peripheral veins.
5. Low measured blood pressure and urine output.

Causes

1. Hypovolaemia, due to intra-operative haemorrhage or pre-existing fluid deficits.
2. Peripheral vasodilation, following general anaesthesia, epidural anaesthesia, most pre-anaesthetic and anaesthetic agents, endotoxaemia or anaphylaxis.
3. Myocardial depression, from pre-existing heart disease, general anaesthetics, hypoxia or ischaemia, 'toxaemia' or electrolyte disturbance.
4. Disturbance of the cardiac rate and rhythm such as sinus bradycardia, atrio-ventricular block, premature ventricular complexes or ventricular tachycardia.
5. Failure of venous return due to vascular obstruction such as pericardial effusions, tumours around or within the great veins or atria, improper surgical packing or increased intrathoracic pressure such as positive pressure ventilation or tension pneumothorax.
6. Reflex hypotension, especially in the case of mesovarium and coeliac manipulation.

Management

Treatment should be directed at the principal cause of the hypotension.

1. Lighten the plane of anaesthesia and discontinue surgical manipulation.
2. Control haemorrhage, use a slight head-down tilt and administer intravenous fluids rapidly (see chapter 15).
3. Give 100% oxygen if this is not already being used.
4. Treat any cardiac arrhythmias. Bradycardia and atrio-ventricular block can be treated with atropine if it is vagal in origin. If no response is obtained then an isoprenaline infusion (0.2 mg in 500 mls NaCl I/V to effect) can be used. Premature ventricular complexes and ventricular tachycardia can be treated with lignocaine (1–2 mg/kg I/V). In dogs this can be repeated safely should the arrhythmia recur. In cats, propranolol may be used (0.04 mg/kg slowly I/V).
5. Relieve mechanical factors hindering venous return.
6. Vasopressors are not frequently indicated but a phenylephrine infusion (10 mg in 500 ml NaCl I/V to effect) may be used to overcome overwhelming vasodilation. A positive inotrope such as dobutamine (50 mg in 500 ml NaC1 I/V at 2–5 μg/kg/min) can be used to treat myocardial failure.

CARDIAC ARREST

Acute failure of cardiac function.

Signs.
1. No heart beat, pulse or bleeding from surgical sites.
2. Respiratory arrest. (May be 'agonal' breathing).
3. Centrally fixed eye with widely dilated pupils and no palpebral or corneal reflexes.
4. Grey, cyanosed or white mucous membranes. (Note: CRT may be prolonged, normal or shortened).

Causes
1. Hypoxia/Hypercarbia.
2. Electrolyte abnormalities (especially hyperkalaemia).
3. Acidosis.
4. Acute hypotension.
5. Hypothermia.
6. Autonomic nervous system imbalance.
7. Anaesthetic overdosage.
8. Anaesthetic sensitisation of the myocardium to catecholamines, (xylazine, halothane).
9. Pre-existing heart disease.

Management

This is an acute emergency and treatment must be prompt. Emergency oxygenation of the vital organs is the first priority. Establishing a normal heartbeat is the next priority.

You must establish cerebral perfusion within 3 minutes. Stop anaesthetic administration, note the time and call for help immediately.

1. Ensure an open **airway** by using an endotracheal tube.

2. Start **positive pressure ventilation** using an anaesthetic circuit, Ambu bag or the operator's own expirate.
   Initially, give 3-4 breaths rapidly, followed by 10-12 breaths per minute, synchronised with external cardiac compression.

3. Begin **cardiac compression/massage.**
   a. External cardiac compression in most adult dogs is performed in right lateral recumbency with a sandbag located beneath the heart. Using the palm of the hand, pressure is applied to the left costochondral junctions which lie over the heart. In barrel chested breeds, however, dorsal recumbency with pressure applied to the sternum may give better results. In puppies and cats, effective compression can be achieved by exerting pressure with the thumb and forefingers on each side of the thorax. Use a rate of 60-80 compressions per minute, with compression occupying 50% of the cycle. Synchronise compressions with ventilation. If you are single handed, it is more important to maintain cardiac compressions than to ventilate, therefore, give two breaths after each 15 compressions. If there is more than one person, give a breath about every five compressions, thus:

	Compressions	Breaths
One person	15	2
More than one person	5	1

   Monitor the effectiveness of external technique by assessing:
       i. the femoral pulse
       ii. mucous membrane colour, and
       iii. the degree of pupillary dilation

   If no improvement is being achieved, alter the technique or consider the possibility of open chest cardiac massage.

- b. Open chest cardiac massage is performed when the chest is already open or when external cardiac massage is ineffective. An emergency thoracotomy is performed through the fifth or sixth intercostal space. There is not time for an aseptic technique. Avoid cutting the intercostal or internal thoracic arteries. Once the heart is exposed, gently massage it from apex to base between the fingers and the palm of one hand. Take care to avoid puncturing a ventricle or interfering with a major thoracic or coronary blood vessel.
- c. The effectiveness of cardiac compression/massage can be improved by:
    - i. a 30° head-down tilt to improve venous return,
    - ii. rapid administration of intravenous fluids (up to 90 mls per kg per hour), and
    - iii applying a pressure bandage around the abdomen.

4. **Drug therapy** initially comprises adrenaline and sodium bicarbonate.
    - a. Adrenaline is used to stimulate sinus rhythm, increase contractility and constrict the peripheral vasculature. Take 1 ml of 1:1000 adrenaline and dilute in 9 mls of sterile water. Give 1 ml per 10 kg (0.01 mg/kg) intravenously or intracardiac if the heart is exposed. Repeat every 10 minutes during arrest.
    - b. Sodium bicarbonate is used to treat acidosis. Give 1 mEq/kg (ie 1 ml/kg of 8.4% $NaHCO_3$) intravenously if resuscitation is longer than 5 minutes or if acidosis before the arrest is suspected. Repeat at 10 minute intervals.

5. **Evaluation** of the cardiac rhythm is now necessary if a normal sinus rhythm has not been established. Three types of condition are commonly seen, and each requires different treatment.
    - a. Ventricular asystole (no electrical activity). Repeat treatment with adrenaline, and sodium bicarbonate as necessary. In addition, give atropine sulphate (0.04 mg/kg I/V) if vagal tone is thought to be increased.
    - b. Electromechanical dissociation (almost normal ECG, no mechanical activity). If adrenaline and sodium bicarbonate are ineffective, give calcium gluconate (20 mg/kg I/V) or calcium chloride (5 mg/kg I/V).
    - c. Ventricular fibrillation (electrical chaos in the ventricles). See below.

6. **Fibrillation therapy.** If ventricular fibrillation is present in spite of good oxygenation, cardiac massage, and treatment with adrenaline and sodium bicarbonate, specific steps have to be taken to overcome it. Both electrical and chemical methods of ventricular defibrillation have been described.
    - a. Electrical defibrillation by direct current countershock (D.C.C.) is the best means of treatment. However, caution is necessary. Ensure,
        - i. the user's hands are dry,
        - ii. all monitors have been disconnected,
        - iii. no-one is in contact with the patient during defibrillation.

      External defibrillation is performed with the electrodes applied directly across the chest. Liberally smear the electrodes with conductive gel and use a setting of between 25 and 100 watt-seconds. Increase incrementally until a response is obtained.

      Internal defibrillation is performed by cradling the heart in specially designed paddles using saline-soaked sponges to ensure a good contact. Use 0.2–0.4 watt-seconds per kg.
    - b. Chemical defibrillation has a much poorer response. Two forms have been shown to be effective.
        - i. Potassium chloride (1 mEq/kg I/V) and acetylcholine (6 mg/kg I/V).
        - ii. Potassium citrate (1 mEq/kg I/V).

      Other drugs are recommended but have no proven efficacy.
        - i. Lignocaine (without adrenaline) (1–2 mg/kg I/V or I/C).
        - ii. Procainamide (2–5 mg/kg slowly I/V).

7. **Follow up therapy** is essential to support the resuscitated heart and to prevent C.N.S. complications from occurring. The following recommendations are suggested.

   a. Respiratory support by continued ventilation and oxygen supplementation until the animal has recovered.

   b. Cardiac support using chronotropic drugs (isoprenaline infusion) where there is bradycardia or inotropic drugs (dobutamine infusion) where there is reduced cardiac contractility.

   c. Blood pressure support by myocardial stimulation (see b.), fluid therapy or vasopressors (phenylephrine infusion).

   d. C.N.S. resuscitation should start immediately with diuretic administration (frusemide 2.5 mg/kg I/V or mannitol 1 gram per kg slowly I/V), steroids, oxygenation and ventilation.

OTHER PROBLEMS

VOMITING AND REGURGITATION

Active or passive reflux of oesophageal or stomach contents into the pharynx with the risk of aspiration.

Signs.

1. Presence of vomitus in the mouth or pharynx (not always visible).
2. Where aspiration has occurred, cyanosis, dyspnoea and tachycardia, will be seen. The sequel to this will be severe, acute pneumonia.

Causes.

1. Presence of stomach contents due to recent feeding or prolonged gastric emptying time.
2. Dilated oesophagus, due to either a vascular ring anomaly or a foreign body.
3. Increased gastric pressure, following surgical manipulation or positioning.
4. Certain anaesthetic drugs, for instance ether, morphine or xylazine.
5. Animals with conditions predisposing them to vomiting, such as gastritis, oesophagitis or intestinal obstruction.

Prevention

1. Pre-anaesthetic fasting; 6 hours is adequate, 12 hours is better if there is delayed gastric emptying.
2. Antiemetic premedication with phenothiazines or butyrophenones.
3. Induced emesis, using morphine or apomorphine.
4. Rapid induction and/or intubation technique. Use intravenous induction agents with the patient in sternal recumbency and with the head elevated. Intubate the trachea and inflate the cuff before placing the animal in lateral recumbency.

Management

1. Removal of vomitus. Immediately position animal in sternal recumbency and lower head to allow the drainage of regurgitated material away from the pharynx. Where suction apparatus is available, remove any vomitus promptly.
2. Aspiration of vomitus. Administer oxygen to prevent hypoxia. Where bronchospasm is present, use aminophylene, diprophylline or etamiphylline (all at 5 mg/kg I/V), pethidine (1–2 mg/kg I/V) or an isoprenaline infusion. Steroids and broad spectrum antibiotics should also be given. Tracheobronchial lavage with saline may be used but it may lead to further spread of vomitus. This should only be performed where suction is available, with the animal in a head down position and preferably with the aid of a bronchoscope.
3. Persistent vomiting in the recovery period can be treated with metoclopramide (0.5 mg/kg I/V).

HYPOTHERMIA

Signs

1. Lowered measured body temperature.
2. Delayed recovery from anaesthesia and a deep plane of anaesthesia when 'normal' clinical dosages are being used (<96 degrees C).
3. Eventually (<96 degrees C), respiratory depression and bradycardia occur.

Causes

1. Reduced thermoregulation while anaesthetised.
2. Evaporative losses, through respiratory system (especially when non-rebreathing systems are in use), surgical preparation or open body cavities.
3. Conduction, convection and radiation, due to cold surfaces and/or cold rooms. Small animals are more susceptible due to their high surface to volume ratio.
4. Administration of cold fluids either I/V or for lavage.

Prevention

1. Insulation, using blankets, various packaging materials, 'Vet Bed' or 'bubble' packaging material.
2. Supplementary heat, raise the ambient temperature to 22°C, use electric or water heating pads (38°C), heating lamps or hot water bottles.
   TAKE CARE! Overzealous heating can cause severe burns.
3. Careful surgical preparation. Clip and cleanse as small an area as is consistent with adequate asepsis, so as to avoid wetting patient excessively.
4. Warm fluids to 37°C before administration.
5. Keep anaesthesia time as short as possible, especially in small patients with open body cavities.

Management

1. Insulate the patient, provide additional heat and finish the procedure as soon as possible (see above).
2. Reduce the administration of anaesthetics. The potency of anaesthetics is markedly potentiated by hypothermia.
3. Where severe hypothermia is present, use only warm intravenous infusions and warm intraperitoneal lavage fluids.

Table 16.1
Suggested Contents of an Emergency Resuscitation Box

Airway and Ventilation
    Ambu bag.
    Face masks: 1 small, 1 medium.
    Laryngoscope with small and medium blades.
    Endotracheal tubes: 3.5, 5.0, 7.0, 9.0, 11.0 and 14.0, internal diameter, all cuffed.
    Tracheotomy tube.

Venous Access/Administration
    Syringes: 2 x 20 ml, 3 x 10 ml, 5 x 5 ml, 5 x 2 ml.
    Needles: 20 x 20G.
    Butterfly needles: 2 x 21G, 2 x 23G.
    Catheters: 2 x 18G, 2 x 20G, 2 x 23G.
    Three-way tap/Intermittent injection caps.
    Fluid administration set.

Surgical Cut Down/Thoracotomy
    Surgical spirit, antiseptic skin preparation.
    A sterile pack consisting of: scalpel handle and blades, rat-tooth forceps,
    tissue forceps, 2 pairs of artery forceps, scissors, gauze swabs and suture material.

Miscellaneous
    Scissors, cotton wool, 1" gauze bandage.
    Gauze swabs, 1" zinc oxide tape.

Drugs
    Adrenaline 1:1000 (5 x 1 ml ampoules).
    Aminophylline, diprophylline or etamiphylline.
    Atropine 0.6 mg/ml (1 x 25 ml vial).
    Calcium gluconate 10% (2 x 10 ml ampoules).
    Doxapram 20 mg/ml (1 x 20 ml vial).
    Isoprenaline 0.2 mg/ml (2 x 1 ml ampoules).
    Lignocaine 20 mg/ml (without adrenaline) (1 x 50 ml vial.).
    Metoclopramide 5 mg/ml (1 x 2 ml ampoules).
    Naloxone 0.4 mg/ml (3 x 1 ml ampoules).
    Sodium bicarbonate 8.4% (1 x 50 ml vial).
    Sodium chloride 0.9% (1 x 500 mls).

Table 16.2
Drugs Commonly Used During a Resuscitation Attempt

Drug	Indications	Dosage and Administration
Adrenaline 1:1000 (1 mg/ml)	Ventricular asystole Ventricular fibrillation Electromechanical dissociation	0.01 mg/kg I/V or I/Cardiac (I/C). (Dilute 1 ml 1:1000 adrenaline in 9 mls water for injections; give 1 ml/10 kgs)
Atropine (0.6 mg/ml)	Bradycardia Atrioventricular block Before neostigmine	0.04 mg/kg I/V or I/M.
Aminophylline (250 mg/ml) Diprophylline (250 mg/ml) Etamiphylline (140 mg/ml)	Bronchoconstriction Left ventricular failure	2.5 mg/kg slowly I/V or I/M. I/V administration should proceed slowly over a 5 minutes period. Etamiphylline should be diluted with an equal volume of water for injections before administration.
Calcium gluconate (100 mg/ml)	Electromechanical dissociation	20 mg/kg slowly I/V or I/C.
Dobutamine (250 mg)	Myocardial failure	2–5 μg/kg by I/V infusion. (Add 50 mg to 500 mls NaCl: give 0.5–1.0 ml/20 kg/min I/V).
Doxapram (20 mg/ml)	Respiratory depression	1.1 mg/kg I/V or sub-lingual. Repeat after 15 mins if needed.
Frusemide (50 mg/ml)	Diuresis Cerebral oedema	2.5 mg/kg slowly I/V.
Isoprenaline (0.2 mg/ml)	Bradycardia Atrioventricular block Bronchoconstriction	Add 1 ml (0.2 mg) to 500 mls NaCl (0.4 μg/ml). Infuse to effect.
Lignocaine (20 mg/ml)	Premature ventricular complex Ventricular tachycardia	1–2 mg/kg I/V. Repeatable in dogs. Not repeatable in cats without side effects.
Mannitol (500 mg/ml)	Cerebral oedema	1.0 gram per kg slowly I/V.
Metoclopramide (5 mg/ml)	Persistent vomiting	0.5 mg/kg I/V, I/M, S/C.
Naloxone (0.4 mg/ml)	Opioid induced respiratory depression	10–20 μg/kg I/V. Repeatable every 15 minutes if needed.
Neostigmine (0.5 mg/ml)	Respiratory depression due to non-depolarising muscle relaxants	0.05 mg/kg slowly I/V. Preceeded by atropine (0.04 mg/ml).
Pethidine (50 mg/ml)	Bronchoconstriction	2 mg/kg slowly I/V.
Phenylephrine (10 mg/ml)	Acute vasodilation	Add 1 ml (10 mg) to 500 mls NaCl (20 μg/ml). Infuse to effect.
Sodium Bicarbonate (84 mg/ml)	Metabolic acidosis	Give 1 mEq/kg slowly I/V (ie 1 ml/kg of the 8.4% solution).

CHAPTER 17

ANAESTHESIA OF EXOTIC SPECIES

J. E. Cooper B.V.Sc., Cert. L.A.S., D.T.V.M., M.R.C.Path., F.I.Biol., F.R.C.V.S.

INTRODUCTION

In view of the wide range of animals which are to be considered, ranging from primates to invertebrates, emphasis in this chapter will be laid on general principles and species' differences. It should be stressed from the outset that to cover (for example) 'bird anaesthesia' or 'reptile anaesthesia' in a few paragraphs, is as unsatisfactory as devoting an equivalent amount of space to 'mammal anaesthesia'. Reference should, therefore, be made to the publications listed for more detailed information about particular species. Anaesthetic techniques are dealt with adequately in earlier Sections.

Euthanasia of exotic species is not covered; in the majority of cases an overdose of a suitable anaesthetic agent is both satisfactory and humane. (Conversely, low doses of certain injectable agents may cause sedation or tranquillisation). Euthanasia may be necessary in order to prevent unnecessary pain, discomfort or distress: this humanitarian aspect must not be neglected, even in apparently less sensitive groups of animals. Analgesia is similarly important; there is published information on pain relief in mammals (see, for example, Flecknell, 1987) but not generally in other groups.

Background information about 'exotic' species is available in standard works (e.g. Cooper and Hutchison, 1985; Fowler, 1986; Poole 1987).

EQUIPMENT

Certain equipment is of particular value when anaesthetising non-domesticated animals and the main items in this category are:-

Anaesthesia chamber.

This is of use in a wide variety of species (Cooper and Hutchison, 1985; Applebee and Cooper, 1989). Ideally, it is attached to an anaesthetic machine and the gases/volatile liquids passed through it; however, it can also prove successful if an appropriate inhalation agent (preferably methoxyflurane, which will not usually reach high and potentially dangerous concentrations) is introduced on a piece of cotton-wool placed in the chamber. If the latter technique is used, the cotton-wool should either be enclosed in a small piece of wire gauze or placed beneath a grid floor in the chamber so as to prevent the animal from coming into contact with volatile liquid.

A suitable anaesthetic chamber for small rodents, cagebirds and reptiles is shown below.

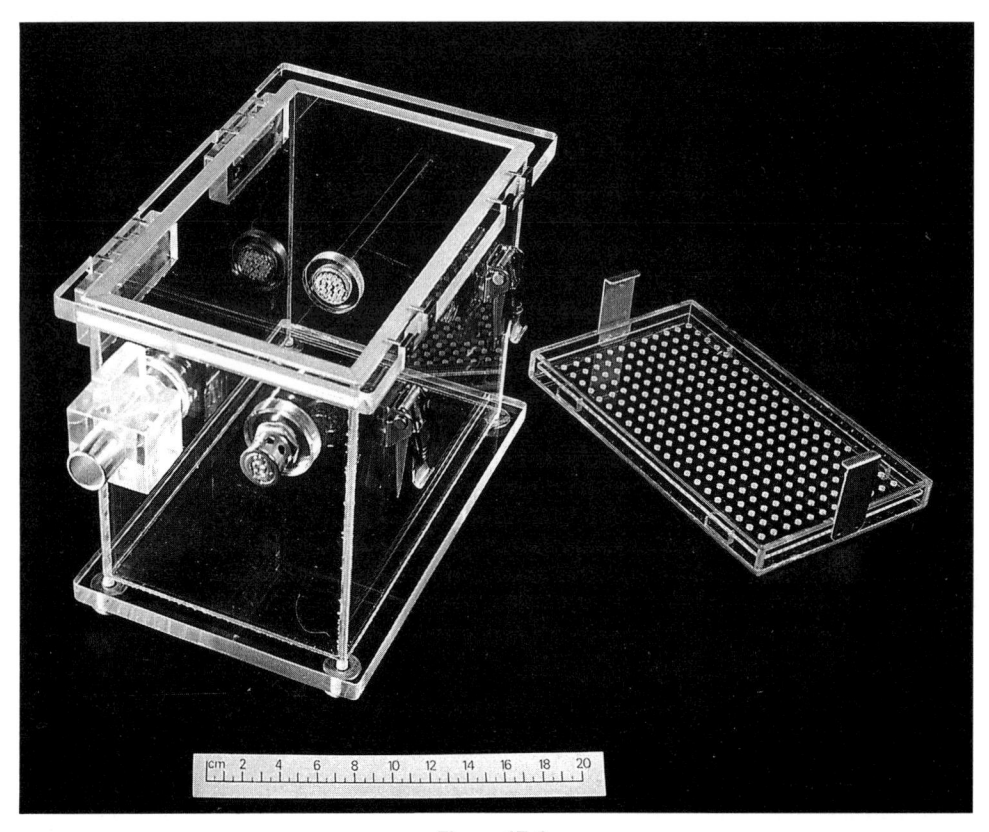

Figure 17.1
Anaesthetic chamber.
The perforated tray on the right permits urine to drain and keeps the animal dry.

The chamber should be made of glass or a suitable transparent plastic so that the animal can be observed from all sides. By carefully tilting the chamber the presence or absence of a righting reflex (see later) can be assessed without opening the lid.

Under practice conditions it is often possible to make a satisfactory chamber from existing materials — for example, a plastic ice-cream container, although this lacks the advantage of visibility. With this and other non-glass containers care must always be taken to ensure that volatile agents, especially ether, do not damage the constituent material. When anaesthetising invertebrates, small glass bottles or vials are useful; the gas or volatile agent can be passed through tubing into these containers.

Canvas or cloth bags.

These bags, which should have a string or tape round the neck, are ideal for weighing small animals (see later). In addition they can, if suspended away from solid objects, make useful 'recovery bags'; a small bird, for example, can flap in such a bag without damaging itself.

Spring balance.

A small animal can be best weighed by placing it in a bag and using a spring balance or accurate electronic scales. Various types of spring balance are available; ideally the veterinary surgeon should have two — one weighing up to 100 grammes, the other up to 1000 grammes.

Small syringes and needles.

1 ml and 0.5 ml syringes are needed routinely, although smaller ones (for example, 0.25 ml), are also of value. 25, 26 or 27 gauge needles are used regularly in work with small animals.

Monitoring equipment.

Careful monitoring of anaesthesia will minimise deaths and emergencies. The Imp respiratory monitor and the Silogic heart monitor are used by the author in a variety of exotic species.

In the case of other equipment, improvisation is often necessary. For example, endotracheal tubes for small birds and mammals can be fashioned from drip tubing or catheters; facemasks can be made from plastic syringe containers.

GENERAL CONSIDERATIONS

As with other species, familiarity with a particular method of anaesthesia is of the utmost importance (Green, 1979). The agents listed in this Section are recommended but the exclusion of others does not necessarily mean they are unsuitable. The veterinary surgeon who feels confident with a particular method should not, so long as it is humane, feel obliged to change it.

The main groups of animals to be discussed are the mammals, birds, reptiles, amphibians, fish and invertebrates. It cannot be over-emphasised that, zoologically speaking, these animals differ greatly. For example, only the first two are 'homeothermic' or 'endothermic' (warm blooded), the others being 'poikilothermic' or 'ectothermic' (cold blooded). As a result, it is vital that the veterinary surgeon wishing to anaesthetise an unusual species should acquaint himself with its natural history and characteristics. Only in this way will he be able to restrain the animal adequately, choose an anaesthetic technique and cope with emergencies. Nevertheless, comparable methods can often be used with different species and, where this is the case, information will not be duplicated.

The general rules of anaesthesia are applicable to non-domesticated species (Green, 1979). Particular care must always be taken when anaesthetising sick or debilitated animals and careful pre-operative examination is important.

Small mammals and birds, which tend to have a high metabolic rate, should not be deprived of food for more than three hours before anaesthesia and water must be provided until the induction of anaesthesia or pre-anaesthetic medication. As a general rule, the larger the animal the longer the period of fasting necessary. Lower vertebrates should be starved for at least 24 hours and, in the case of snakes and other species which swallow whole prey, for 4-5 days. Invertebrates should not, in general, be starved but those species which take blood, eg. leeches and ticks, may regurgitate if they have recently fed.

In all species balanced anaesthesia, using two or more agents, is usually preferable to the administration of large doses of one drug.

MONITORING

The assessment of depth of anaesthesia can pose problems in many of the species discussed in this chapter. In the case of mammals, standard methods (as used in domesticated species) are usually applicable. In other groups, the pattern of reflexes is different and less reliable as indicators. The use of dissociative agents eg. ketamine, will further complicate the situation. Respiratory rate and response to pressure or pain are helpful guidelines in birds. Response to pressure or pain is also reliable in lower vertebrates. The presence or absence of a righting reflex (when the animal is put on its back) is a useful guide as to when a potentially dangerous animal, such as a venomous snake, can be safely handled. Many of the ectothermic (cold blooded) species appear very resistant to hypoxia and therefore should not be assumed dead because of a total absence of response. Exposure to air or oxygen, especially with assisted positive pressure ventilation or the use of a respiratory stimulant eg. doxapram, will often result in the restoration of respiration and total recovery.

POST-OPERATIVE CARE

Such features as post-operative care and maintenance of fluid balance are important in all species though there are few scientific data on these in the lower vertebrates or invertebrates. Maintenance of a normal body temperature is especially relevant to small mammals and birds. In the case of ectotherms the general rule, pending proper research, is to maintain the animal at its preferred body temperature, especially in the recovery stage.

The duration of anaesthesia is not usually stated in the subsequent pages, partly because it can depend upon the dose but mainly on account of the considerable variation between species. Small birds and mammals tend to metabolise drugs rapidly and therefore the effects of most injectable agents pass off within 1-1 ½ hours. Lower vertebrates, on the other hand, may (especially if they are temperate species kept at a low temperature) take several hours to recover from comparable doses of the same agent. Even recovery from inhalation agents may be delayed in certain species — for example in snakes, where a reservoir of anaesthetic agent can remain in the animal's air sac unless flushed out with oxygen. These variations make post-operative care of the greatest importance and any animal which appears to be taking a long period to recover should be subjected to intensive care, including monitoring (see earlier).

ANAESTHETIC AGENTS

In the succeeding pages, doses of anaesthetic agents are given in mg (or ml) per kilogramme of body weight. This is usually satisfactory in practice but ideally doses should be scaled allometrically (Cooper and Hutchison 1985, Kirkwood, 1983) to make allowance for different metabolic rates.

There are six agents or combinations of agents that are particularly valuable in 'exotic' animals and which will be listed frequently in the subsequent pages.

These are:-

Ketamine hydrochloride 'Ketalar', 'Vetalar', (Parke-Davis), or 'Ketaset', (C-Vet) by injection (usually intramuscular but occasionally intravenous). There is some doubt as to whether this dissociative agent is, strictly, an anaesthetic but clinical experience suggests that it produces a reasonable degree of analgesia in certain species eg. primates. It is often preferable to use it at a low dose to quieten or immobilise the animal and then to deepen or maintain anaesthesia with an inhalation agent. The addition of other injectable drugs may potentiate the effect of ketamine and enhance its effect — for example intraperitoneal or intramuscular diazepam 'Valium', (Roche) or midazolam 'Hypnovel', (Roche) will improve muscle relaxation and promote a smoother recovery, while xylazine 'Rompun', (Bayer) may enhance analgesia.

The veterinary preparation of ketamine contains 100 mg/ml: for small animals it is more satisfactory to use the human (paediatric) concentration of 10 mg/ml or 50 mg/ml 'Ketalar' or to dilute 'Vetalar' with normal sterile saline.

Following intramuscular administration of ketamine, the duration of sedation/anaesthesia is usually 20-40 minutes. There is considerable species variation but the animal will generally recover completely within two hours. Lower vertebrates are an exception and may remain sedated for up to 24 hours.

Alphaxalone-alphadolone 'Saffan', (Pitman-Moore) by intramuscular or intravenous injection. This drug will produce light to medium surgical anaesthesia on its own but, like ketamine, can also be used in combination with an inhalation agent. Alphaxalone-alphadolone is a viscous solution and care must be taken not to draw too many air bubbles into the syringe. There is also a tendency for the syringe to become sticky and for the needle not to fit tightly.

Intramuscular alphaxalone-alphadolone usually produces sedation/anaesthesia of 30-50 minutes duration, with total recovery within three hours. In the case of intravenous administration the figures are 10-15 minutes and one hour respectively.

Halothane and oxygen by inhalation. Although not specifically mentioned in the text, the addition of nitrous oxide ($N_2O:O_2$ at a ratio of 1:1) is to be commended, particularly in view of its analgesic and muscle relaxant properties. Induction can sometimes be carried out adequately using a facemask or anaesthetic chamber but in either case consideration has to be given to the question of human safety because of halothane in the environment. Often it is preferable to employ an injectable agent initially and then intubate. 4% halothane is usually best for induction, 1—2% for maintenance.

Isoflurane is attracting increasing attention and proving useful in a wide range of species: it can be used in a similar way to halothane but tends to produce a more rapid induction and recovery and has a higher safety margin.

Methoxyflurane and oxygen by inhalation. This combination is excellent for a wide range of species, including poor risk patients such as wild birds. Induction is slow but safe and there is post-operative analgesia. Again, the addition of nitrous oxide is usually advisable especially since this will help to deepen anaesthesia.

Fentanyl-fluanisane 'Hypnorm', (Janssen Pharmaceutals). This neuroleptanalgesic is particularly valuable in small mammals (not felids). Muscle relaxation is enhanced if it is supplemented with midazolam 'Hynovel', (Roche): the two can be mixed together in a syringe or a 'cocktail' can be prepared.

A point should be made about local analgesia. In the case of the mammals, local analgesics can be employed in a similar way to domestic species. Details are therefore not given. Local analgesics are **not** recommended in birds other than ethylchloride as a spray or, in the larger (over 1000 g) birds only, a diluted (0.1–0.2%) solution of lignocaine. Products containing adrenaline should not be used. In reptiles and amphibians local analgesic agents can be employed as in mammals but with caution; again, a 0.1–0.2% solution is probably advisable. Local analgesia is not recommended in fish or invertebrates.

GROUPS OF ANIMALS

PRIMATES

Small species of monkey, such as the common marmoset (*Callithrix jacchus*) and squirrel monkey (*Saimiri sciureus*) are not uncommonly kept as pets. All primates except marmosets are covered by the Dangerous Wild Animals Act (Cooper, 1987).

General Points.

Primates should be handled with care in view of the possible dangers of zoonoses: protective clothing is essential. A crush cage is useful for restraint; nets and bags will also be needed. Adequate physical restraint is essential before inducing anaesthesia: one should not attempt to handle primates weighing over 5 kg single handed. These animals have great strength for their size and many, especially males, have large canine teeth. Intramuscular injections should be given into a limb, using as small a needle as practicable. Maintenance of body temperature and fluid balance during and after anaesthesia is particularly important.

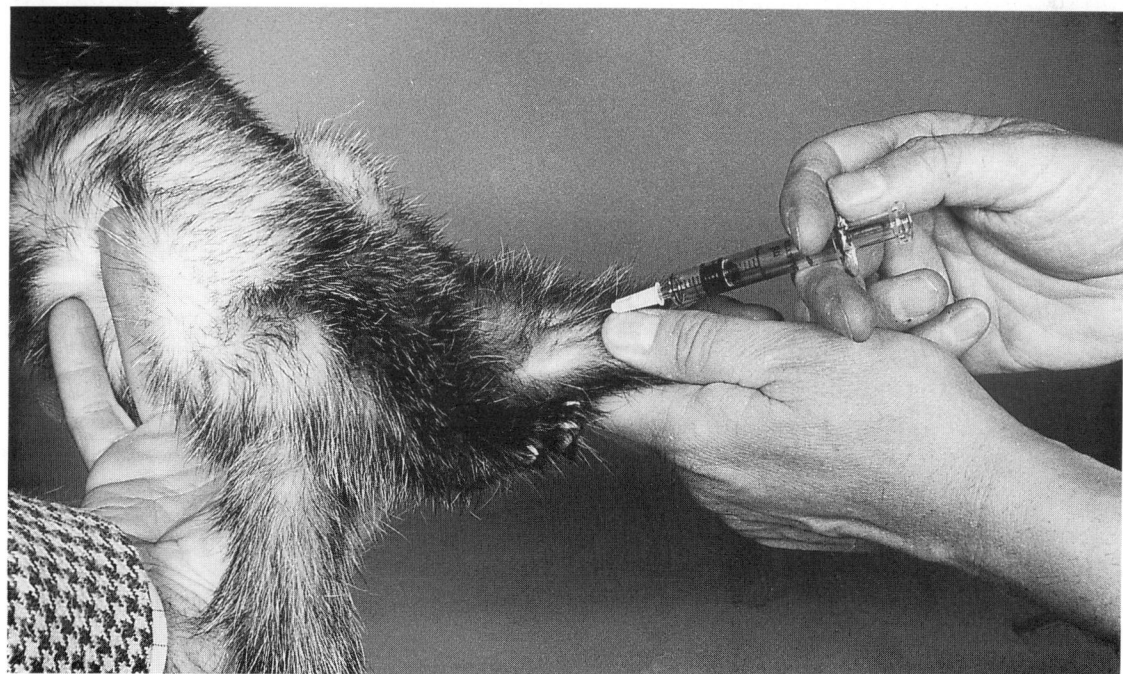

Figure 17.2
Intramuscular injection of ketamine in the hindleg of a ferret.
Note that the animal has to be held firmly in order to minimise struggling.

Methods of anaesthesia
  Ketamine by I/M injection 10–50 mg/kg, preferably supplemented with I/M midazolam 0.5 mg/kg.
  Alphaxalone-alphadolone by I/M injection 8–25 mg/kg.
  Halothane (or isoflurane) and oxygen by facemask or endotracheal tube.
  Methoxyflurane and oxygen as above.

CARNIVORES

These primarily include the ferret (*Mustela putorius furo*) and mink (*M. vison*), both members of the Family Mustelidae. Other small carnivores can usually be dealt with in a similar manner.

General Points.

Handle with care to avoid bites; a ferret can usually be grasped round the neck with thumb under its jaw but the body must be supported. Intramuscular injections should be given into the hind leg (Cooper, 1985).

Methods of anaesthesia
  Ketamine by I/M injection 10–30 mg/kg, preferably supplemented with midazolam 0.5–2 mg/kg or xylazine 1 mg/kg.
  Alphaxalone-alphadolone by I/M injection 6–15 mg/kg.
  Halothane (or isoflurane) and oxygen by inhalation.
  Methoxyflurane and oxygen by inhalation.

LAGOMORPHS

These comprise the rabbit *(Oryctolagus cuniculus)* and hare *(Lepus europaeus)*.

General Points.

These animals should be handled carefully since lagomorphs can kick strongly with their hindlegs and spinal damage may result. Wrapping the animal firmly in a towel will help, as may covering the eyes. Intravenous injections are best given into the marginal vein of the ear after shaving the hair and applying spirit; warming the ears will help to dilate the veins. A 'butterfly' attachment to the syringe will reduce the risk of the needle coming out of the vein if the animal moves its ear. For intramuscular injections the hind leg should be used.

Barbiturates must only be used with great caution in lagomorphs and it should be noted that the high incidence of upper respiratory disease in rabbits can make anaesthesia hazardous. Premedication with doxapram (0.25 ml/kg I/M) will help to reduce the risk of respiratory failure.

Methods of anaesthesia
  Fentanyl-fluanisone by I/M injection 0.25 ml/kg. Anaesthesia can be deepened with an intravenous or inhalation agent.
  Alphxalone-alphadolone by I/V injection 5–15 mg/kg.
  Halothane (or isoflurane or **methoxyflurane)** and oxygen by inhalation.
  Methohexitone sodium 'Brietal', (Elanco) by I/V injection 5–10 mg/kg.
  Ketamine by I/M injection 25 mg/kg plus xylazine I/M (or small incremental doses I/V).
  Propofol 'Rapinovet', (Coopers) appears useful by I/V injection 10 mg/kg and may prove safer and more reliable than alphaxalone-alphadolone.

RODENTS

The majority of the small mammals seen in veterinary practice fall into this group. Common examples are the mouse (*Mus musculus*), rat (*Rattus norvegicus*), Mongolian gerbil or jird (*Meriones unguiculatus*) and guinea pig (*Cavia porcellus*).

General Points.

Although all closely related, the small rodents have many different characteristics, some of which may influence anaesthesia (Flecknell, 1985, 1987). For example, most have a high metabolic rate and as result tend to absorb, metabolise and excrete agents rapidly. While the majority have a tail which can be used in handling and for intravenous injections, the guinea pig does not.

More specifically, different strains of mice and rats may react differently to the same agent. The anaesthetic methods listed below are applicable to many species but particular note should be taken of specific contra-indications. An anaesthetic chamber is of great value when dealing with rodents but they can also be intubated: an auroscope will facilitate this.

Methods of anaesthesia

Fentanyl-fluanisone by I/M injection 0.5 ml/kg (should be supplemented with I/M diazepam or midazolam 2.5 mg/kg in guinea pigs and mice).

Methoxyflurane and oxygen by inhalation.

Halothane (or isoflurane) and oxygen by inhalation.

Ketamine by I/M injection 10—50 mg/kg (of limited value only, poor in mice and rats; only valuable for non-painful procedures in guinea pigs).

BIRDS

Birds vary in size and shape. Those most commonly seen in veterinary practice include the budgerigar *(Melopsittacus undulatus)* and other psittacine birds, canary *(Serinus canaria)*, British (cage or aviary-bred) passerines, foreign passerines, birds of prey and pigeons (Coles, 1985). In addition, advice may be sought on any species of wild bird found as a casualty (Cooper, 1975; Cooper & Eley, 1979).

General Points

Small birds have a high metabolic rate and a high (approximately 41°C) body temperature; as a result drugs are metabolised rapidly and the maintenance of warmth during anaesthesia is particularly vital.

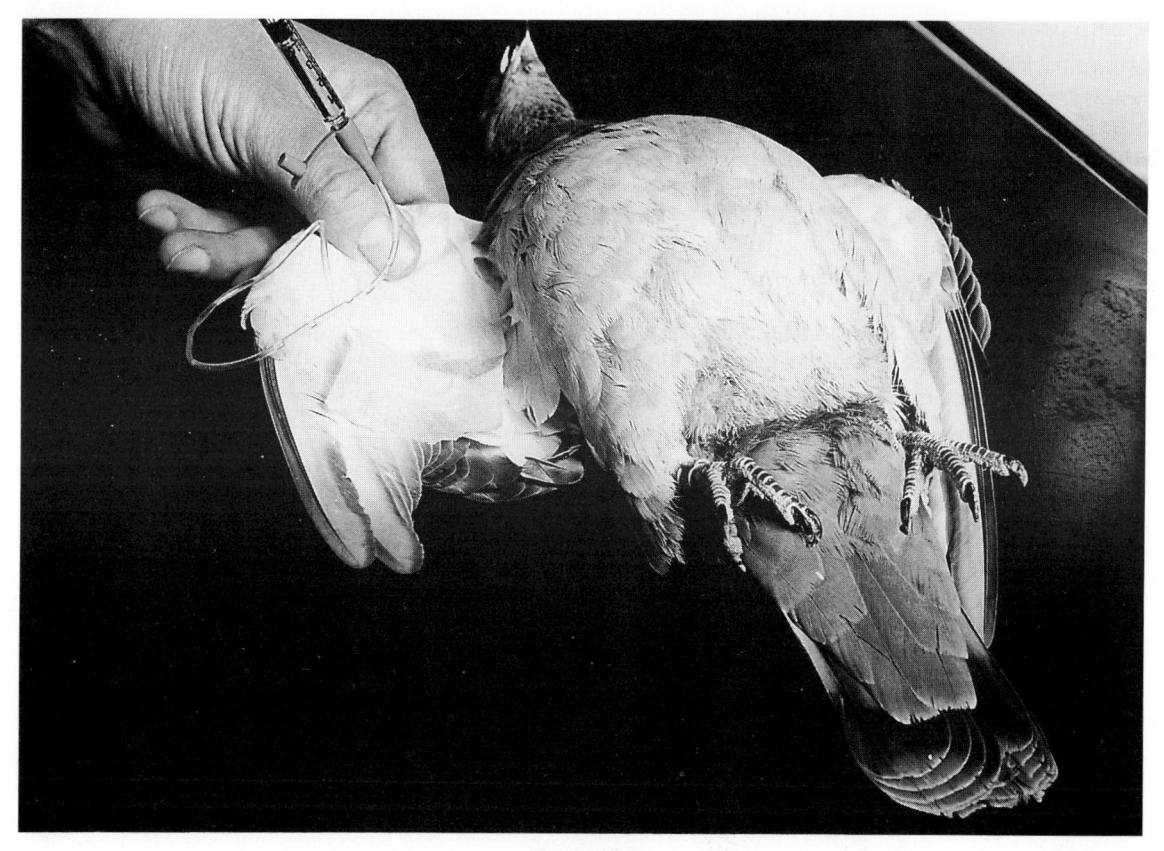

Figure 17.3
Maintenance of intravenous anaesthesia in a pigeon. A butterfly attachment permits incremental doses (in this case of methohexitone) to be given in the brachial (basilic) vein. The needle is lightly held in place with a piece of white tape.

Birds are easy to intubate; the glottis lies at the base of the tongue and is readily visible. For intravenous injections either the brachial (basilic) vein, which crosses the ventral surface of the radius and ulna just distal to the elbow joint, or the tarsal vein, which runs across the anterior surface of the leg, should be used. Intramuscular injections can be given into the pectoral or leg muscles; there is less danger of impairing flight if the latter are used. An anaesthetic chamber is useful for small birds.

Methods of anaesthesia

Ketamine by I/M injection 5—50 mg/kg combined with other agents (eg. midazolam) where appropriate.

Alphaxalone-alphadolone by I/V injection 2—10 mg/kg or by I/M injection 35 mg/kg.

Propofol by I/V injection 3—5 mg/kg, with incremental doses as necessary.

Halothane (or isoflurane) and oxygen by inhalation.

Methoxyflurane, nitrous oxide and oxygen by inhalation.

REPTILES

Many species of reptile may be presented for veterinary attention, mainly lizards, snakes, tortoises and terrapins (Cooper & Jackson, 1981; Frye, 1981; Marcus, 1981). Crocodilians (crocodiles, alligators, caimans, etc.) are less often seen, but can be anaesthetised in a similar way to large lizards.

General Points

Reptiles should be handled with care and, in the case of poisonous snakes, advice and assistance should be sought from someone with experience. Some non-poisonous species, such as pythons and monitor lizards, reach a large size and must also be handled with caution. All reptiles are ectothermic (cold blooded) and therefore their metabolic rate — including body temperature and response to drugs — is likely to be related to the ambient temperature. This can have a marked influence on the induction, maintenance and recovery from anaesthesia. Reptiles are often relatively resistant to hypoxia: this is particularly marked in terrapins. Reptiles are easy to intubate as the glottis lies well forward. Intravenous injections are not difficult (although there can be species and individual variation); in snakes and lizards the tail vein is approached from the ventral surface, in chelonians from the dorsum. For intramuscular injections the legs can be used (lizards, chelonians and crocodilians) or the dorsal or lateral musculature (snakes and legless lizards). It is often easier, and is usually perfectly satisfactory, to inject snakes subcutaneously; the site is on the side of the body with the needle pointing towards the snake's head. Reptiles are very prone to bacterial infection; prior cleaning of the skin with alcohol or povidone-iodine is therefore desirable. An anaesthetic chamber is useful for small species.

Methods of anaesthesia

Alphaxalone-alphadolone by I/V injection 9 mg/kg or I/M 15 mg/kg (not in terrapins).

Ketamine by I/M injection 10—50 mg/kg with or without supplementation with an inhalation agent. This is often not satisfactory in chelonians but is a useful technique in snakes and lizards.

Halothane (or isoflurane) and oxygen by inhalation.

Methoxyflurane and oxygen by inhalation.

Propofol is also proving useful by I/V injection 1.0—1.4 ml/kg (M.P.C. Lawton, personal communication).

Hypothermia (30 minutes at 4°C) can be used to quieten a reptile but is of limited value and under no circumstances should it be considered a humane anaesthetic technique.

AMPHIBIANS

Many species of frog, toad, newt and salamander are kept as pets, in zoological collections and for scientific study (Nace *et al*, 1974). Some, such as the clawed frog *Xenopus* spp., are maintained in large numbers in research institutes.

General Points.

Amphibians have moist skins and must not be allowed to become too dry or hot. Anaesthetic and surgical techniques are best performed with the animal wrapped in a damp cloth. Thin rubber gloves may facilitate handling and will reduce the risk of skin irritation from the parotid secretion of toads (Cooper, 1985).

Like reptiles, amphibians are ectothermic. In addition, immature amphibians breathe through gills and even adults can respire to a certain extent through the skin. Because of the thin skin, drugs (including anaesthetics) can be absorbed into the bloodstream from the water.

Intubation of the larger species is possible. The technique used is comparable to that in reptiles.

Intramuscular injection can be given into the hind leg but spirit should not be used to clean the site. Drugs can be injected by the subcutaneous route (under the skin over a limb) and are rapidly absorbed.

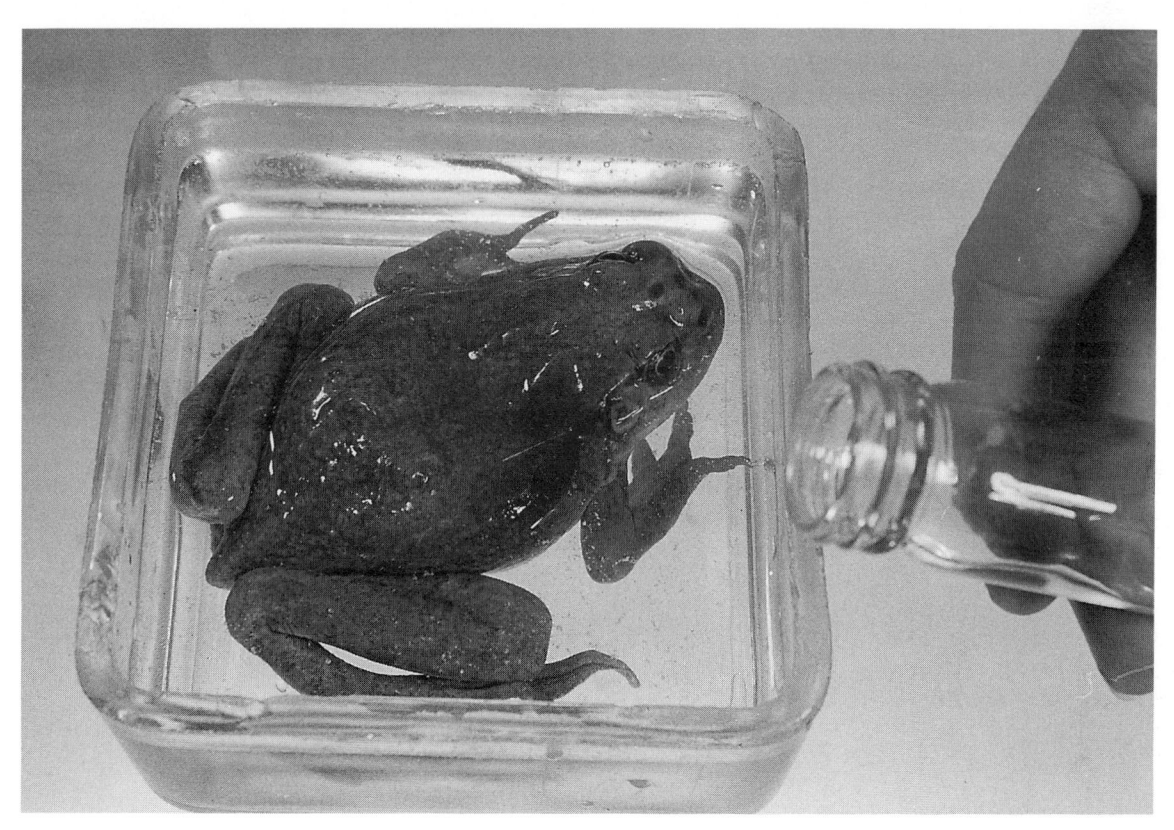

Figure 17.4
A frog is anaesthetised prior to surgery
The animal is placed in a chamber containing water to which benzocaine, dissolved in acetone, is being added.

Methods of anaesthesia

Ketamine by I/M injection 25–50 mg/kg.

Halothane (or isoflurane) and oxygen by inhalation.

Methoxyflurane and oxygen by inhalation.

Tricaine methanesulphonate 'MS 222', (Sandoz) by absorption; the agent is appropriately diluted in water (usually 1/2000–1/3000) into which the amphibian is placed. This method is ideal for immature gill-bearing amphibians but less satisfactory (and slower) in adults. Care must be taken to ensure that adult animals do not inhale water; they should be anaesthetised in a shallow bowl which enables them to keep their nostrils in the air. Conversely, larval amphibians must not be kept **out** of water for more than five minutes. Anaesthesia is reversed by placing the animal in fresh water. 'MS 222' is a powder which must be kept cool and in the dark. Freshly prepared solutions should be used.

Benzocaine (BDH Laboratories) by absorption — 1/5,000–1/10,000 dilution: the benzocaine is first dissolved in acetone.

Hypothermia — see reptiles.

FISH

The veterinary surgeon may be approached over tropical or temperate fish of either freshwater or marine species (Scott, 1985). Some of these are kept as pets or for display, some for research and some for food. Their rquirements differ considerably.

General Points.

The vast majority of fish are entirely aquatic and should be handled as little as possible. Once removed from the water they must be kept moist, in a damp net or cloth. Damage to the skin surface can result in fluid and electrolyte imbalance and predispose to infection. Like reptiles and amphibians, fish are ectothermic. However, many are very sensitive to sudden fluctuations in temperature and therefore care should be taken to maintain them within their optimum range. Injectable agents can be given into the muscles at the base of the tail but most anaesthetics are administered in the water; the fish absorbs the agent through the gills. Recovery takes place when the fish is returned to its own tank or to a container of "clean" water.

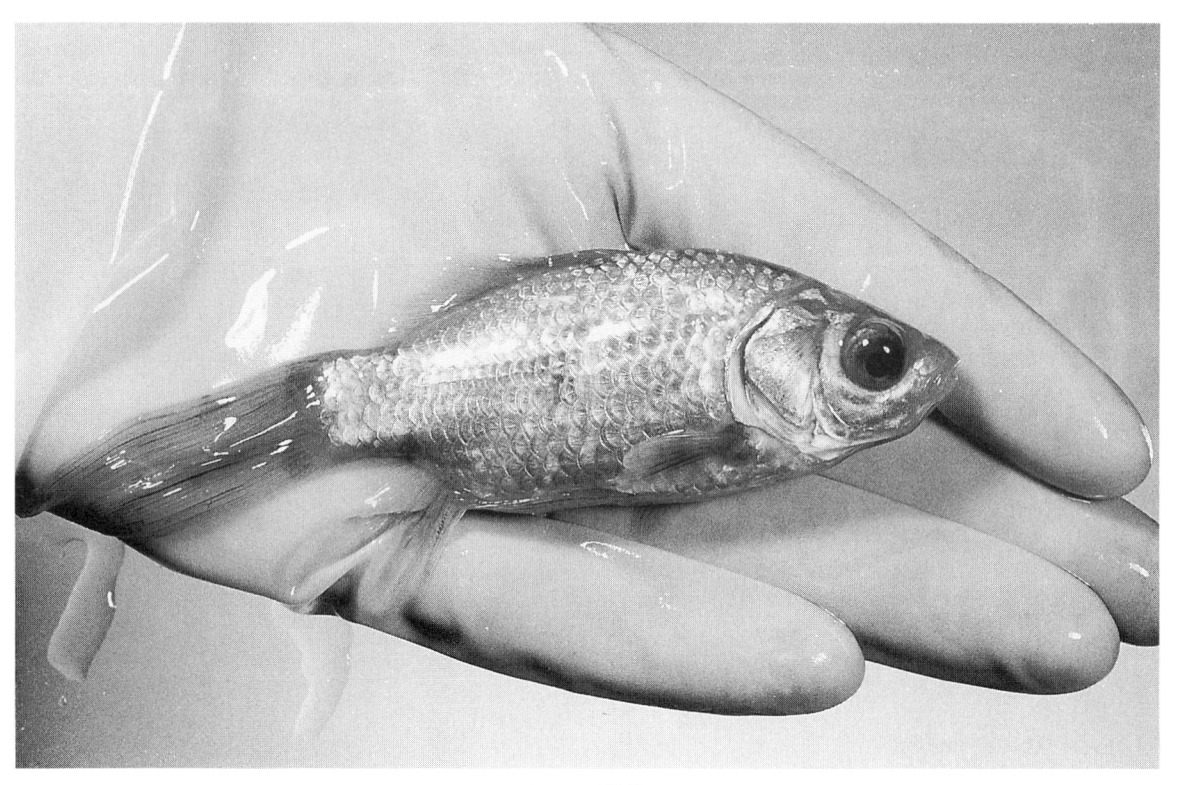

Figure 17.5
A live fish with a bacterial infection (note the petechiae on the fins) is examined in the hand.
Light anaesthesia with benzocaine or tricaine methanesulphonate will permit this to be carried out efficiently and humanely.

Methods of anaesthesia

Tricaine methanesulphonate 'MS 222' by absorption through the gills. The concentration used depends upon the species, its size and the temperature. It is often wise to use a 1/40,000 dilution for an initial trial.

Benzocaine (in acetone) by absorption — 1/10,000 — 1/40,000 dilution.

Halothane or other inhalation agents by absorption 2—3 ml per litre of water.

Please note

Ethyl carbamate (urethane) should **not** be used as it is a carcinogen. In an emergency carbon dioxide (provided from a cylinder or by the addition to the tank of small quantities of soda water) can be employed.

INVERTEBRATES

The invertebrates either have no skeleton or (for example, insects and crustaceans) have a tough, external skeleton composed of chitin (Cooper, 1980, 1985). Some species are entirely aquatic, others terrestrial. Some have limbs, some do not.

General Points.

Relatively little is known of the ability of invertebrates to feel pain and they are excluded from the provisions of the Animals (Scientific Procedures) Act 1986 which controls experiments on animals. Nevertheless, research on some species has revealed that their nervous system is remarkably complex and every effort should therefore be taken to reduce the risk of causing unnecessary pain or discomfort. Unfortunately, little work has been carried out on anaesthesia, even by laboratories specialising in these animals, and therefore the methods listed below, while of value in immobilising the invertebrates, may not produce analgesia.

Methods of anaesthesia

Ether, halothane or carbon dioxide by inhalation (terrestrial species).

Tricaine methanesulphonate 'MS 222' or **benzocaine** in acetone by absorption (aquatic species). Similar dilutions are used to those recommended for fish. A mixture of pentobarbitone and 'MS 222' has proved particularly useful in snails (Mutani, 1982).

Carbon dioxide by absorption (aquatic species). The gas can be bubbled through the water or soda water may be added.

Hypothermia (30 minutes at 4°C) is commonly used to immobilise or to slow the response of invertebrates. However, although nerve conduction is retarded, there is no evidence that this produces analgesia. In the case of terrestrial and freshwater molluscs the use of cooled boiled water, from which air has been excluded, has been recommended; the animals are placed in this overnight.

Acknowledgements

I am grateful to P. A. Flecknell, M. P. C. Lawton, A. W. Sainsbury and B. M. Q. Weaver for reading and commenting upon this chapter.

REFERENCES AND FURTHER READING

GENERAL

(These cover more than one group or general principles and are particularly recommended for the veterinary surgeon who deals with a variety of species.)

APPLEBEE, K. and COOPER, J. E. (1989). An anaesthetic or euthanasia chamber for small animals. *Journal of Animal Technology.* (not yet published).

COOPER, J. E. and BEYNON, P. H. (1991). Editors, *Manual of Exotic Pets.* BSAVA, Cheltenham.

COOPER, M. E. (1987). *An Introduction to Animal Law.* Academic Press, London.

FOWLER, M. E. (1974). Restraint and anesthesia in zoo animal practice. *J. Am. vet. med. Ass.* **164**, 176.

FOWLER, M. E. (1986). *Zoo and Wild Animal Medicine.* 2nd ed. W. B. Saunders, Philadelphia.

GREEN, C. J. (1979). *Animal Anaesthesia.* Laboratory Animals, London.

HARTHOORN, A. M. (1975). *The Chemical Capture of Animals.* Ballière Tindall, London.

JONES, D. M. (1977). The sedation of birds and reptiles. *Vet. Rec.* **101**, 340.

JONES, D. M. (1976). Recent advances in the use of drugs for immobilisation, capture and translocation of non-domestic animals. *Veterinary Annual* **16**, 280.

KIRKWOOD, J. K. (1983). Dosing exotic species. *Vet. Rec.* **112**, 486.
POOLE, T. B. (1987). Editor, *The UFAW Handbook on the Care and Management of Laboratory Animals.* 6th ed. Longman, Essex.
STUNKARD, J. A. and MILLER, J. C. (1974). An outline guide to general anesthesia in exotic species. *Vet. Med. /Small Anim. Clin.* **69**, 1181.

MAMMALS

BOX, P. G. and ELLIS, K. R. (1973). Use of CT1341 anaesthetic (Saffan) in monkeys. *Lab. Anim.* **7**, 161.
BREE, M. M., FELLER, I. and CORSSEN, G. (1967). Safety and tolerance in repeated anaesthesia with C1 581 (ketamine) in monkeys. *Anaesthesia and Analgesia* **46**, 596.
COOPER, J. E. (1991) Ferrets. In *Manual of Exotic Pets.* (See General Section).
FLECKNELL, P. (1991). Guinea pigs, rabbits and rats and mice. In *Manual of Exotic Pets.* (See General Section).
FLECKNELL, P. (1987). *Laboratory Animal Anaesthesia.* Academic Press, London.
GREEN, C. J. (1975). Neuroleptanalgesic drug combinations in the anaesthetic management of small laboratory animals. *Lab. Anim.* **9**, 161.
GREEN, C. J. (1978). Anaesthetising ferrets. *Vet. Rec.* **102**, 269.
GREEN, C. J., KNIGHT, J., PRECIOUS, S. and SIMPKIN, S. (1981). Ketamine alone and combined with diazepam or xylazine in laboratory animals: a 10 year experience. *Lab. Anim.* **15**, 163.
MACKINTOSH, C. J., MACARTHUR, J. A., LITTLE, T. W. A. and STUART, P. (1976). The immobilisation of the badger (*Meles meles*). *Brit. vet. J.* **132**, 609.
PHILLIPS, I. R. and GRIST, S. M. (1975). Clinical use of CT 1341 anaesthetic (Saffan) in marmosets (*Callithrix jacchus*). *Lab. Anim.* **9**, 57.

BIRDS

CAMBURN, M. A. and STEAD, A. G. (1978). Anaesthesia in wild and aviary birds. *J. small Anim. Pract.* **19**, 395.
COLES, B. H. (1985). *Avian Medicine and Surgery.* Blackwell, Oxford.
COOPER, J. E. (1975). First aid and veterinary treatment of wild birds. *J. small Anim. Pract.* **16**, 579.
COOPER, J. E. and ELEY, J. T. (1979). Editors. *First Aid and Care of Wild Birds.* David and Charles, Newton Abbott.
COOPER, J. E. (1978). *Veterinary Aspects of Captive Birds of Prey.* Standfast Press, Glos.
COOPER, J. E. and FRANK, L. (1973). Use of the steroid agent CT1341 in birds. *Vet. Rec.* **92**, 474.
HAIGH, J. C. (1981). Anaesthesia of raptorial birds. In *Recent Advances in the Study of Raptor Diseases.* (eds. Cooper, J. E. and Greenwood, A. G.). Chiron, Keighley.
HARCOURT-BROWN, N. H. (1978). Avian anaesthesia in general practice. *J. small Anim. Pract.* **19**, 573.
HARRISON, G. J. and HARRISON, L. R. (1986). Editors. *Clinical Medicine and Surgery.* W. B. Saunders, Philadelphia.

REPTILES

COOPER, J. E. (1974). Ketamine hydrochloride as an anaesthetic for East African reptiles. *Vet. Rec.* **95**, 37.
COOPER, J. E. and JACKSON, O. F. (1981). Editors. *Diseases of the Reptilia.* Academic Press, London.
FRYE, F. L. (1981). *Biomedical and Surgical Aspects of Captive Reptile Husbandry.* Veterinary Medicine Publishing Co., Kansas.
JACKSON, O. F. and LAWRENCE, K. (1991). Chelonians. In *Manual of Exotic Pets.* (see General Section.)
LAWRENCE, K. (1991). Lizards and snakes. In *Manual of Exotic Pets.* (see General Section.)
LAWRENCE, K. and JACKSON, O. F. (1983). Alphaxalone-alphadolone anaesthesia in reptiles. *Vet. Rec.* **112**, 26.
MARCUS, L. C. (1981). *Veterinary Biology and Medicine of Captive Amphibians and Reptiles.* Lea and Febiger, Philadelphia.

AMPHIBIANS

COOPER, J. E. (1991). Amphibians. In *Manual of Exotic Pets.* (See General Section).

NACE, G. W., CULLEY, D. D., EMMONS, M. V,, GIBBS, E. L., HUTCHINSON, V. H. and MACKINNELL, R. G. (1974). *Amphibians — guidelines for the breeding, care and management of laboratory animals.* Inst. Lab. Anim. Resources, Nat. Acad. Sci., Washington D.C.

FISH

HARVEY, B., DENNY, C., KAISER, S. and YOUNG, J. (1988). Remote intramuscular injection of immobilising drugs into fish using a laser-aimed underwater dart gun. *Vet. Rec.* **122**, 174.

JOLLY, D. W., MAWDESLEY-THOMAS, L. E. and BUCKE, D. (1972). Anaesthesia of fish. *Vet Rec.* **91**, 424.

SCOTT, P. W. (1991). Ornamental fish. In *Manual of Exotic Pets.* (See General Section).

STUART, N. C. (1981). Anaesthesia in fishes. *J. small. Anim. Pract.* **22**, 377.

INVERTEBRATES

ASHBURNER, M. and WRIGHT, T. R. F. (1978). The laboratory culture of Drosophila. In *The Genetics and Biology of Drosophila.* (eds. Ashburner, M. and Thompson, J. N.). Academic Press, London.

COOPER, J. E. (1980). Invertebrates and invertebrate disease; an introduction for the veterinary surgeon. *J. small Anim. Pract.* **21**, 495.

COOPER, J. E. (1991). Invertebrates. In *Manual of Exotic Pets.* (See General Section).

DEMERC, M. and KAUFMAN, B. P. (1973). *Drosophila Guide, 8th ed.* Carnegie Institute, Washington.

MEYER, H. U. (1957). Obtaining completely relaxed and stretched live larvae of D. melanogaster. *Drosophila Information Service.* **31**, 176.

MUTANI, A. (1982). A technique for anaesthetising pulmonate snails of medical and veterinary importance. *Zeitschrift für Parasitenkunder.* **68**, 117.

RUNHAM, N. W., ISANKURA, K. and SMITH, B. J. (1965). Methods for narcotising and anaesthetising gastropods. *Macologia.* **2**, 231.

APPENDIX

J. F. R. Hird, M.A., B.V.Sc., D.V.A., M.R.C.V.S.
M. H. Clark, B.Sc., B.Vet.Med., M.R.C.V.S.

THE CONTROL OF OPERATING THEATRE POLLUTION BY GASEOUS AND VOLATILE ANAESTHETICS

INTRODUCTION: THE NEED FOR ACTION

In 1967 a paper suggested that prolonged exposure to anaesthetic gas pollution might be harmful. Further studies suggested that the effects might include an increased spontaneous abortion rate, infertility, increased incidence of congenital abnormalities in children of exposed staff, and impaired motor skills, perception and memory.

Nitrous oxide is additionally known to inhibit cobalamine and prevent the normal synthesis of folate. Daily exposure to it is known to produce a condition resembling pernicious anaemia in experimental animals and has been widely used by research haematologists. Exposed rats show an increased incidence of foetal abnormalities; the minimum concentration required is probably 800 to 1000 ppm over a period of several hours per day. Epidemiological surveys in exposed human subjects have failed to demonstrate such a definite relationship. This is probably because such subjects were exposed near the lower limit of the danger zone, and it is no cause for complacency.

Halothane has not been shown to cause physical danger to staff in human operating theatres. However, those are usually large and well ventilated, with well maintained equipment and specialist anaesthetists. This is seldom true of veterinary theatres. Ether is potentially explosive and is assigned an occupational exposure standard (OES) of 400 ppm.

The Health and Safety Executive (HSE) definitely regards anaesthetics as substances hazardous to health within the remit of the COSHH regulations. A practice's COSHH assessment of its use of these agents should therefore include both the precautions to be taken to limit exposure to safe levels, **and the means of determining whether safe levels are in fact achieved.** The importance of monitoring was emphasised by a survey within the BSAVA North East Region. Personal dosemeters were used to measure the average concentrations to which surgeons and anaesthetists were exposed during an operating session. The results ranged from below 5 ppm to over 1000 ppm. These results compare with a 'target' level of 100 ppm, and a probable limit of 250 ppm to be set by HSE. Some of the practices with high levels were using active scavenging apparatus. The possession and use of such equipment does not guarantee safety. To keep theatre pollution levels low, careful attention has to be paid to equipment **and** technique.

TYPES OF SCAVENGING SYSTEM

1. Passive
The simplest system consists of a length of 22mm clear plastic scavenging tubing connected to the scavenge valve of the anaesthetic circuit. This is led outside the building. It is only suitable for use where an outside wall lies within 8' of the circuit. Even then, the pipework presents significant resistance and the breathing circuit may be affected by wind pressure from outside the building. There are many situations in which the scavenging efficiency of these systems will prove unsatisfactory. The HSE is unlikely to be convinced.

2. Active – Passive
As above, but discharging into a forced ventilation duct rather than directly outside. Could be useful where the layout of the theatre allows for short pipework, but few veterinary practices rely on powered ventilation.

3. Activated Charcoal Absorbers
These suffer from three major disadvantages. First, they do not remove nitrous oxide, which is the most important pollutant. Second, they are a passive system with an increased resistance, and third, they can continue in use when the absorbent is 'full' and no longer working.

4. Active Systems
Can be installed in any operating theatre irrespective of its position. Suitably designed, they can be made completely efficient. They are more expensive to install, but will probably prove to be the only system which will satisfy the requirements of HSE in years to come.

THE DESIGN OF ACTIVE SCAVENGING SYSTEMS

Within NHS hospitals, theatres are now equipped with scavenging systems to BS 6834. Briefly, this specifies a high capacity pump connected to the patient's expiratory valve by a receiver. This receiver is an air break device, carefully designed to prevent too great a suction being applied to the patient whilst simultaneously having sufficient capacity to prevent a suddenly exhaled tidal volume from escaping into the theatre. The receiver designed at Barnsley General Hospital is now in common use. It incorporates various fail safe devices and a silencing mechanism. Air suction devices can be noisy.

This approach to scavenging technique requires a pump capable of moving volumes of air several times greater than the minute volume of the patient. Experience has shown that some active scavenging systems available on the veterinary market use too small a pump to work effectively.

PERSONAL EXPOSURE MONITORING

Whatever scavenging technique is used, HSE will expect practices to have assessed its effectiveness. HSE itself has plans to measure nitrous oxide exposure of staff in veterinary practices in 1992, so this is of immediate importance. Infrared imaging of nitrous oxide clouds within theatres has shown that general room levels of the gas are irrelevant. What matters is the personal exposure of the staff, particularly the anaesthetist and surgeon. This can be measured.

Personal dosemeter tubes about the size of a fountain pen are worn as near to the face as is convenient. These are prefilled with an absorbent. At the end of one wear period (an operating session of a couple of hours) they are resealed and returned to the monitoring service. The absorbed gas is driven off by heat and measured by gas chromatography. The dosemeter tube can be re-used.

If satisfactory results are achieved during a typical operating session, there is no need for continuous monitoring. Monitoring should be repeated after any change in operating theatre design, anaesthetic equipment or technique. Scavenging systems must be checked every 14 months (HSE requirement). Provided all the equipment is correctly maintained and used, personal exposure should remain acceptable. Occasional monitoring would emphasise the need for staff to follow good practice and guard against unobserved equipment malfunction.

When oxygen/nitrous oxide/halothane mixtures are administered, the halothane cannot exceed a certain fixed proportion of the nitrous oxide. It follows that, if the nitrous oxide pollution falls within acceptable levels, the halothane must also. Practices using nitrous oxide do not, then, need to monitor their halothane pollution separately. This is sufficiently well documented that HSE will accept it. However, practices which do not use nitrous oxide will need to show that their halothane levels are acceptable. Halothane exposure is measured in exactly the same way as nitrous oxide, although the demands of calibration mean that the two substances cannot be run through the same apparatus simultaneously. Although ether could be similarly measured, in practice the demand for personal ether monitoring is nonexistent and no service is readily available. In any case, the 400 ppm limit for ether relates more to its inflammability, and therefore to general room levels. These can be measured by infrared absorption.

ACCEPTABLE LEVELS OF PERSONAL EXPOSURE

At the time of writing, only ether has its OES of 400 ppm. However, it is very probable that the HSE will fix a limit for nitrous oxide of 250 ppm, as an 8 hour time weighted average (TWA). Sweden has fixed a limit of 100 ppm 8 hr TWA for nitrous oxide. This has been shown to be achievable in hospitals and the preliminary results of the BSAVA NE survey showed approximately half of the participants doing even better. There is presently no limit set for halothane.

PRACTICAL WAYS TO REDUCE ANAESTHETIC POLLUTION

Switching on an active scavenging system does not guarantee low personal exposure. Unless it is used with real care, it may induce a false sense of security. All staff must be instructed and motivated to achieve the lowest possible levels of pollution.

1. Unless the connection between the patient and the anaesthetic apparatus is gas tight (leaks, masks, cuffed endotracheal tubes) large leakages can occur. None of these will be scavenged.
2. The patient must be connected to the circuit before nitrous oxide or other anaesthetics are switched on.
3. Nitrous oxide and other anaesthetics must be switched off **and the breathing system purged with fresh oxygen** to force anaesthetics along the scavenging system before the patient connection is broken.
4. Periodic monitoring should be used to check effectiveness and reinforce the need for constant care.

KENNELS AND RECOVERY AREAS

Many practices are forced, through lack of an alternative, to site recovery areas in cellars and other places with unsatisfactory natural ventilation. During recovery the inhaled agents are exhaled, polluting this part of the workplace. Some practices may feel the need to provide additional forced ventilation and monitor staff working in recovery areas.

ACKNOWLEDGEMENTS
We would like to acknowledge that this article could not have been written without the enthusiastic assistance of Dr. John O'Sullivan, principal pharmacist, and Dave Gill, senior hospital engineer, of Barnsley District General Hospital.

INDEX

ABC maintenance 20, 23
Acepromazine 41–2, 48, 90, 103, 108
Accidents, anaesthetic 129–37
Acupuncture 10
Adrenaline 75, 102, 133, 137, 143
Alcuronium 84
Alfentanyl 115
Alpha 2 Adrenoceptor Agonists 43–4
    Antagonists 44-45, 131
    combinations 46-47
Alphaxalone/Alphadolone Acetate ('Saffan')
    55–6, 91, 108, 115, 117, 142
Amethocaine 77
Aminophylline 130, 134, 137
Amphibians 143, 146–7
Anaemia 19
Anaesthetic risk (USA) 17
Analgesia/analgesics 23, 33–7, 40, 115, 139
    epidural 87–8
    local 11, 37, 75–81, 102–3, 143
Antibiotics 19
Anticholinergic drugs 90, 108, 110, 115
Anticonvulsive therapy 19
Apnoea 130–1
Arterial blood pressure monitoring 22
Atipamezole 44-45
Atracurium 84
Atropine 40, 90, 102, 131, 137

Barbiturates 52–5
Benzodiazepine Antagonists 45, 90, 115
Beta blockers 19, 102
Birds 141–3, 145–6
Blood in fluid therapy 124
Blood gas, pH and electrolyte
    measurement 22
Bupivacaine 37, 77
Buprenorphine 35
Butorphanol 36
Butyrophenones 42–3, 134

Caesarian section anaesthesia 12, 87–92
Calcium gluconate 137
Carbon dioxide 68, 148
Cardiac
    disease 18
    glycosides 19
    problems 131–4
Carnivores 144
Chest drainage 98
Cocaine 75, 76
Cold blooded/warm blooded animals 141
Colloids in fluid therapy 124
Corticosteroids 19, 102, 130
Cremophor EL 11, 55
Crystalloids in fluid therapy 124

Depth of anaesthesia 21
Detomidine 44
Diazepam 44–5, 90, 115–16, 142
Diethyl ether 66
Diprenorphine 36, 131
Diprophylline 130, 134, 137
Dissociative agents 57–9, 141, 142
Diuretics 102
Dobutamine 134, 137
Doxapram 131, 137, 141
Drugs
    analgesic 33–7
    anticholinergic 90, 108, 110, 115
    in Caesarian section operation 87–92
    and cardiac arrest 133
    choice of 15
    controlled (CD) 34
    for emergency resuscitation 136
    for exotic species 142–9
    for geriatrics 108–9
    in high risk cases 115–17
    in hypothermia 135
    in inhalation anaesthesia 65–8, 72–3
    interactions 19
    in intravenous anaesthesia 52–62
    local analgesic 76–7
    muscle relaxants 83–5
    for neonates/pediatrics 110–11
    in ophthalmic surgery 102–3
    for pre-medication 40
    in respiratory emergencies 130–1
    sedative 41–7
    in thoracic surgery 96–8
    and vomiting/regurgitation 136

Ectothermic/endothermic animals 141
Electrocardiogram monitors 22
Emergency cases 113–17, 129–37
    resuscitation kit 136
Enflurane 67
Epidural analgesia 87–8
Equipment 13–14, 25–32
    emergency resuscitation kit 136
    monitoring 22, 29–30, 32
    for non-domesticated animals 139–41
Etamiphylline 130, 134, 137
Ethyl carbamate 148
Etorphine 131
Euthanasia 139
Exotic species 139–49

Fentanyl 35, 46, 108, 115
    see also Hypnorm
Fish 143, 148
Flow rates 72

Fluid(s)
    imbalances 121—2, 126—7
    monitoring 21—2
    therapy 97, 98, 119—27
Flumazenil 45
Frusemide 137

Gallamine 84
Gas 65
Gases in association with anaesthesia 68
General anaesthesia 10, 88—9, 92, 103, 115—16
General principles of anaesthesia 9—15
Geriatrics 107—9
Glucose in fluid therapy 125
Glycopyrrolate 40, 108
Glycopyrronium 90, 102

Halothane 66, 72—3, 108, 110, 115, 117, 142
Hartmann's solution 119, 125
High risk anaesthesia 113—17
Homeothermic animals 141
Hyoscine 40
Hypnorm 47, 48, 62, 143
Hypotension 131
Hypothermia 12, 97, 135, 146, 149
Hypovolaemia 19

Immobilon S.A. 47, 61
Inhalation anaesthesia 10, 65—73, 104
    practical administration 72—3
    techniques for administration 68—72
Insulin 19
Intermittent positive pressure
    ventilation (IPPV) 96, 97
Intravenous anaesthesia 10, 51—62
Invertebrates 141, 143, 149
Isoflurane 67—8, 108, 110, 115, 142
Isoprenaline 130, 134, 137

Ketamine 37, 57—8, 91, 115, 117, 141—2

Lagomorphs 144
Legislation 9, 34
Lignocaine 76, 81, 110, 133, 137, 143
Liver disease 19
Local anaesthesia/analgesia *see* analgesia
Lower vertebrates 141—2

Mannitol 137
Medetomidine 37, 43—4, 48, 90, 115, 131
Methadone 35
Method, choice of 11—12
Methohexitone 12, 54, 90—1, 103, 108, 110
Methoxyflurane 37, 67, 108, 143
Metoclopramide 134, 137
Midazolam 45, 115, 142, 143
Minute volume 72
Miotics 102
Monitoring 20—2, 141
Morphine 34, 90, 115, 134
Mucous membranes 21
Muscle relaxants 83—5, 91, 97, 104, 111, 131

Nalbuphine 36
Naloxone 36, 115, 131, 137
Narcotic drugs 10, 90
Negligence 9
Neonatal animals 11, 92—3, 109—11
Neostigmine 131, 137
Neuroleptanalgesia 45-46, 88
    combinations 47, 61—2
Neuromuscular blocking agents, *see* muscle relaxants
Nitrous oxide (N_2O) 37, 65, 142—3

NSAIDS (non-steroidal anti-inflammatory drugs) 19, 36, 37
Nursing care 13, 37

Opioids 34—6, 37, 40, 131
    opioid/sedative combinations 45—6
Ophthalmic surgery 101—4
Oxygen 65, 68

Pain perception 9, 33, 149
Pancuronium 84
Papaveretum 35
Parasympathetic antagonists 40
Pediatric animals 109—11
Pentazocine 35
Pentobarbitone 54—5, 108
Pethidine 35, 90, 108, 110, 115—16, 130, 134, 137
Phenothiazines 41—2, 110, 115, 134
    combinations 46
Phenylephrine 134, 137
Plasma in fluid therapy 124
Poikilothermic animals 141
Post-operative care 23, 37, 141—2
Pre-medication 19, 39—40
Pre-operative assessment/care 17—19, 37
Preparation for anaesthesia 12
Prilocaine 77
Primates 142—4
Procainamide 133
Procaine 76
Proparacaine 77
Propofol 12, 59—60, 91, 103, 108, 110, 117
Pulse monitoring 20—1

Radiography 12, 98, 114
    sedation for 48
Recovery area 12
Regurgitation 134
Renal disease 19
Reptiles/amphibians 143, 146
Respiratory
    disease 18
    monitoring 20
    problems 129—31
Resuscitation emergency kit 136
Righting reflex 141
Rodents 144—5
'Saffan' *see* Alphaxalone/Alphadolone
Sedative drugs 40—5
    sedative/opioid combinations 45—6
Snakes 141—2, 146
Sodium bicarbonate 119, 124—5, 133, 137
Steroids 55—6
Suxamethonium 84
Sympathomimetics 102

Temperature monitoring 21, 23
Thiopentone 12, 52—3, 90—1, 103, 108
Thoracic surgery 95—8
Tidal volume 72
Tiletamine 59
Tranquillisers 41—2

Ventilatory inadequacy 130—1
Vercuronium 84
Volatile liquids 66—8
Vomiting 134

Warm blooded/cold blooded animals 141

Xylazine 37, 43, 44, 48, 115, 117, 142

Zolazepam 45

LIST OF B.S.A.V.A. PUBLICATIONS

THE JOURNAL OF SMALL ANIMAL PRACTICE

An International Journal Published Monthly Editor W. D. Tavernor, B.V.Sc., Ph.D., F.R.C.V.S.
Fifteen Year Cumulative Index published 1976
Available by post from: B.S.A.V.A. Administration Office, Kingsley House, Church Lane, Shurdington, Cheltenham, Gloucestershire GL51 5TQ

Manual of Parrots, Budgerigars and other Psittacine Birds
Edited by C. J. Price, M.A., Vet.M.B., M.R.C.V.S.
B.S.A.V.A. Publications Committee 1988

Manual of Laboratory Techniques
New Edition
Edited by D. L. Doxey, B.V.M.&S., Ph.D., M.R.C.V.S.
and M. B. F. Nathan, M.A., B.V.Sc., M.R.C.V.S.
B.S.A.V.A. Publications Committee 1989

Manual of Anaesthesia for Small Animal Practice
Third Revised Edition
Edited by A. D. R. Hilbery, B.Vet.Med., M.R.C.V.S.
B.S.A.V.A. Publications Committee 1992

Manual of Radiography and Radiology in Small Animal Practice
Edited by R. Lee, B.V.Sc., D.V.R., Ph.D., M.R.C.V.S.
B.S.A.V.A. Publications Committee 1989

Manual of Small Animal Neurology
Edited by S. J. Wheeler, B.V.Sc., Cert.V.R., Ph.D., M.R.C.V.S.
B.S.A.V.A. Publications Committee 1989

Manual of Small Animal Dentistry
Edited by C. E. Harvey, B.V.Sc., F.R.C.V.S., Dip.A.C.V.S., Dip.A.V.D.C.
and H. S. Orr, B.V.Sc., M.R.C.V.S., D.V.R.
B.S.A.V.A. Publications Committee 1990

Manual of Small Animal Endocrinology
Edited by M. F. Hutchison, B.Sc., B.V.M.S., M.R.C.V.S.
B.S.A.V.A. Publications Committee 1990

Manual of Exotic Pets
New Edition
Edited by P. H. Beynon, B.V.Sc., M.R.C.V.S.
and J. E. Cooper, B.V.Sc., Cert.L.A.S., D.T.V.M., F.R.C.V.S., M.C.R.Path., F.I.Biol.
B.S.A.V.A Publications Committee 1991

Manual of Small Animal Oncology
Edited by
R. A. S. White B.Vet.Med., PhD., D.V.R.,
F.R.C.V.S., Diplomate, American College of Veterinary Surgeons
B.S.A.V.A Publications Committee 1991

Manual of Canine Behaviour
Second Edition
Valerie O'Farrell, Ph.D., Chartered Psychologist
B.S.A.V.A. Publications Committee 1992

Manual of Ornamental Fish
Edited by R. L. Butcher, M.A., Vet.M.B., M.R.C.V.S.
B.S.A.V.A. Publications Committee 1992

Manual of Reptiles
Edited by P. H. Beynon, B.V.Sc., M.R.C.V.S.,
J. E. Cooper, B.V,Sc., Cert.L.A.S., D.T.V.M., F.R.C.V.S., M.C.R.Path., F.I.Biol.
and M. P. C. Lawton, B.Vet.Med., Cert.V.Ophthol., F.R.C.V.S.
B.S.A.V.A Publications Committee 1992

B.S.A.V.A VIDEO 1 (VHS and BETA)
Radiography and Radiology of the Canine Chest
Presented by R. Lee, B.V.Sc., D.V.R., Ph.D., M.R.C.V.S.
Edited by M. McDonald, B.V.M.S., M.R.C.V.S.
B.S.A.V.A. Publications Committee 1983

An Introduction to Veterinary Anatomy and Physiology
By A. R. Michell, B.Vet.Med., Ph.D., M.R.C.V.S.
and P. E. Watkins, M.A., Vet.M.B., M.R.C.V.S., D.V.R.
B.S.A.V.A. Publications Committee, 1989

Proceedings of the B.S.A.V.A. Symposium "Improved Healthcare in Kennels and Catteries"
Edited by P. H. Beynon, B.V.Sc., M.R.C.V.S.
B.S.A.V.A. Publications Committee 1991

Practical Veterinary Nursing
Second Revised Edition
Edited by C. J. Price, M.A., Vet.M.B., M.R.C.V.S.
B.S.A.V.A. Publications Committee 1991

Practice Resource Manual
Edited by D. A. Thomas, B.Vet.Med., M.R.C.V.S.
B.S.A.V.A. Publications Committee 1992

AVAILABLE FROM BOOKSELLERS

Canine Medicine and Therapeutics
Third Edition
Edited by E. A. Chandler, B.Vet.Med., F.R.C.V.S.,
D. J. Thompson, B.A., M.V.B., M.R.C.V.S.,
J. B. Sutton, M.R.C.V.S.
and C. J. Price, M.A., Vet.M.B., M.R.C.V.S.
Blackwell Scientific Publications 1991

An Atlas of Canine Surgical Techniques
Edited by P. G. C. Bedford, Ph.D., B.Vet. Med., F.R.C.V.S., D.V.Ophthal.
Blackwell Scientific Publications 1984

Feline Medicine and Therapeutics
Edited by E. A. Chandler, B.Vet.Med., F.R.C.V.S.
C. J. Gaskell, B.V.Sc., Ph.D., D.V.R., M.R.C.V.S.
and A. D. R. Hilbery, B.Vet.Med., M.R.C.V.S.
Blackwell Scientific Publications 1985

Jones's Animal Nursing
Fifth Edition
Edited by D. R. Lane, B.Sc., F.R.C.V.S.
Pergamon Press 1989